Perioperative Practice

Case Book

Case Book Series

Perioperative Practice

Case Book

**Edited by
Hannah Abbott and
Stephen Wordsworth**

Mc Graw Hill Education

Open University Press

Open University Press
McGraw-Hill Education
8th Floor
338 Euston Road
London
NW1 3BH

email: enquiries@openup.co.uk
world wide web: www.openup.co.uk

and Two Penn Plaza, New York, NY 10121-2289, USA

First published 2016

A catalogue record of this book is available from the British Library

ISBN-13: 978-0-33-526346-2
ISBN-10: 0-33-526346-1
eISBN: 978-0-33-526347-9

Library of Congress Cataloging-in-Publication Data
CIP data applied for

Typeset by Transforma Pvt. Ltd., Chennai, India
Printed and bound by CPI Group (UK) Ltd, Croydon, CR0 4YY

Fictitious names of companies, products, people, characters and/or data that may be used herein (in case studies or in examples) are not intended to represent any real individual, company, product or event.

Praise Page

"Although clearly targeted at the student Operating Department Practitioner, Abbott and Wordsworth have produced a learning resource that any learner in the perioperative environment will find both informative and a useful learning aid. The editors have set out the twenty patient case studies in a sequence that allows the student to work through them as their course and competence progresses, although students can dip into the case studies in any order that supports their current clinical placement.

The section introducing perioperative care is essential reading for any perioperative practitioner, with an up-to-date introduction to the latest concepts of teamwork and human factors in patient safety. Coupled with the patient-centred focus of the case studies this provides any reader with an understanding of the changing approach to patient care in the perioperative environment."

Bill Kilvington, President, College of Operating
Department Practitioners, UK

"I have read this book several times and found that the chapter contents are excellent. This book will be useful for ODPs and theatre nurses, it will enhance their knowledge and skills and may also enhance their abilities to work in operating departments and care well for patients. The book covers preoperative care, intraoperative care and postoperative care which is essential for all practitioners working in operating departments. The content of this book is very informative and will be of great use to both students and qualified practitioners. I find it very impressive and I envisage it to be very useful to all theatre practitioners!"

Paul Wicker, formerly Head of Perioperative Studies,
Edge Hill University, UK and Visiting Professor,
Nanjing University, China.

Dedication

This book is dedicated to the memory of Chris Reay, a friend and colleague still sadly missed. We are sure that he would have welcomed this text, particularly since in his role he advised and mentored many of the authors who have contributed to the book. Chris was dedicated to developing the ODP profession and passionate about helping others to fulfil their potential. Similarly, we hope that the book also contributes to our collective understanding, as well as being useful to learners at various stages of their personal and professional development.

Contents

Notes on editors and contributors

Hannah Abbott (editor) BSc (Hons), PGCE, PgCert, MSc (Science) (Open), ODP, MCODP, FCODP, QTLS. Associate Professor and Associate Head of School, Allied and Public Health Professions, Birmingham City University.

Professor Stephen Wordsworth (editor) Cert Ed, BA (Hons), PgCert, MSc (Health Care Practice), EdD, ODP, MCODP, FCODP. Deputy Dean, Faculty of Health, Social Care and Education, Anglia Ruskin University.

Ella Davies BSc (Hons), ODP. Physician's Assistant (Anaesthesia) Student, West Suffolk Hospital, Bury St Edmunds, Suffolk.

Karen Evans RGN, Dip HE, BSc (Hons), PgCert, FHEA. Associate Professor, Birmingham City University.

Kelly Goffin Dip HE, BSc (Hons), RN. Clinical Research Nurse, James Paget University Hospitals Foundation Trust.

Katie Hide RN, DPSN, Cert Ed, BSc, MEd, RNT. Lecturer, Plymouth University.

David Hughes MA Ed, PgDip Ed, ODP. Senior Lecturer, Birmingham City University.

Agnes Lafferty MN, PgCert Ed, RNT, BA Nursing Studies, RN. Lecturer, Operating Department Practice, Glasgow Caledonian University, and Charge Nurse, Theatres, Wishaw General Hospital, NHS Lanarkshire.

Melanie Leek RN, Dip HE Nursing Practice, BSc (Hons) Nursing Practice (Adult). Staff Nurse, Ophthalmic Theatres, Ipswich Hospital NHS Trust.

Claire Lewsey MSc, BN, PgCert, RGN, SFHEA. Programme Lead, BSc Operating Department Practice, Glasgow Caledonian University.

Adele Millington RGN, DPSN (Adult), MEd, BSc (Hons) Clinical Nursing Studies (Adult) Perioperative Pathway. Senior Lecturer, Birmingham City University.

Simon Nixon BA (Hons), PgDip, MSc, ODP. Senior Lecturer, Birmingham City University.

Romilly Norman ODP. ODP and Clinical Practice Facilitator, Ipswich Hospital NHS Trust.

Mark Owen ODP, BSc, MSc, FHEA. Professional Lead and Lecturer, Plymouth University.

Sue Parker EdD, MA (Ed), BSc (Open), Cert Ed. Senior Operating Department Practitioner, Education and Quality, University Hospital North Staffordshire.

Mark Ranson MA, FHEA, PGCIHE, BSc (Hons), Specialist Practitioner (NMC), Dip HE, RGN. Senior Lecturer (Acute and Critical Care), University Campus Suffolk.

Fiona Ritchie MSc, PgCert, BSc, RN, FHEA. Lecturer, Department of Nursing and Community Health, Glasgow Caledonian University.

Ray Swann BSc (Hons), MA (Ed), ODP. Senior Lecturer, Birmingham City University.

List of tables

Preface

This book has been written primarily to support pre- and post-registration operating department practitioners (ODPs) in the delivery of holistic, evidence-based care to patients undergoing surgery. This text therefore encompasses all aspects of the ODP role and the core knowledge required for this, however we recognise that this will be equally relevant to perioperative nurses as well as providing a useful resource for perioperative support workers.

As ODPs we are both passionate about the delivery of high-quality care to patients within the perioperative environment, as we recognise the great privilege afforded to us when caring for a patient at their most vulnerable. As part of this role therefore we believe it is essential to understand the perioperative intervention in the context of the patient's wider healthcare experience and psychosocial needs, in order to ensure the patient receives individualised care. It is for this reason that we have adopted a case study approach in this text. While there are many texts that offer an 'instructions'-style approach for perioperative care, these do not enable the reader to apply theoretical principles to individual patients. As the ODP role has evolved, there is an increasing focus on the ODP as an autonomous practitioner who is able to assess, plan and deliver care, and who is accountable for their decision making. It is our intention therefore to demonstrate how a robust knowledge base, in conjunction with an appropriate assessment, can result in the delivery of effective care to a given patient.

We have selected a range of common procedures from a range of surgical specialties, the majority of which will form part of the workload in most local hospitals, and we feel this makes the book valuable to all practitioners. We have also included some more specialist cases to allow the reader to gain an appreciation of specialist clinical settings and how the patient pathway can vary between settings. Within these case studies you will also find a range of patient demographics as well as a range of different clinical techniques, with the intention that this text overall will cover a wide scope of practice. It is not our intention however that you read this text as a single book; rather we hope that you will read the case studies relevant to your practice/development needs at the appropriate time, and we have identified the level of complexity of each case based on the academic year of study. Our decision making regarding which case studies are advised for each academic year is based on the case study as a whole and therefore includes the complexity of the patient and the writing style; therefore you may find some 'routine' cases are perhaps a Year 3 (Level 6) case study, and this may be because the patient has a number of complex physical or psychosocial care needs or because the care has been explored in more detail. Please remember however that these academic years are advisory only, so you shouldn't feel discouraged from reading case studies 'early' if they relate to your current clinical placement, for example.

We would encourage you to reflect upon the care in these case studies as part of your continued development, and we have included some 'Stop and think' boxes to encourage you to consider alternatives or the wider implications of the care. In terms of the language used, you will also find some variation in the tense, with some texts using the future and others the past tense. This is deliberate as we want you, the reader, to think about what care you would plan for the patient (future tense) as well as to reflect on the care delivered (past tense). All case studies include a 'References and further reading' section, which offers a starting point for your own wider reading relating to the topic – although you must remember that practice is evolving continually due to new research, hence you should always search for any updated evidence.

The case studies have been written by ODPs and nurses from academic and clinical settings throughout the country, who are united in their keen interest in perioperative care. The regional variation within the text should be viewed positively as this demonstrates variation in local practice, and it is important to note that there can be a number of variations in the delivery of safe, evidence-based care. This is intended to allow the reader to gain exposure to variations in practice, and we hope it will prompt critical reflection upon your own practice and experience, with consideration of how improvements in care may be achieved. In the same way there are also variations in the writing style throughout, reflecting the varied approaches and philosophies of care planning – for example, some case studies have a medical focus, while others adopt a more social approach. Again, this is intended to allow the reader to appreciate the different approaches to care in a contemporary healthcare setting.

We hope that you will enjoy this book and that you will find it beneficial as you develop in your career within the perioperative environment.

Hannah Abbott and Stephen Wordsworth

Introduction to perioperative care
Hannah Abbott and Stephen Wordsworth

INTRODUCTION TO PERIOPERATIVE CARE

The term 'perioperative' was originally adopted to describe the care within the operating department, however the term literally means 'around the operation', from the Latin 'peri' meaning 'around' (Woodhead and Fudge, 2012). Perioperative care therefore encompasses the complete care of the patient including preoperative assessment and preparation, in addition to the care the patient receives within the operating department. The increasing focus on the principle of holistic care has further extended the scope of perioperative care; it 'describes the care of the patient from the initial referral and diagnosis to full recovery, or as full as that recovery might be for their physical condition' (Woodhead and Fudge, 2012: 3). It is therefore essential that practitioners within the operating department consider the entire patient journey as the decisions made relating to care within the operating department may also impact upon the patient's immediate and long-term recovery.

Perioperative care has changed significantly over the past 15 years; this is due to a number of interrelated factors, including an ageing population, patients with increasing co-morbidities, the greater complexity of interventions involving rapid technological advances and equipment development, the introduction of a range of non-medical roles, and the expansion of the types and location of surgery such as increased day surgery provision. Between 2002/03 and 2012/13 there was a 60% increase in the number of surgical procedures, which in 2012/13 alone resulted in 10.6 million procedures being carried out (NHS Confederation, 2014).

Clearly these factors have the potential to impact on the way that care is delivered within the perioperative environment. Indeed the high stakes and intensity of the environment, in combination with the 'high degree of technical competence that may be required, and the level of pressure the staff experience can make it feel rather clinical, and therefore dispassionate' (Wordsworth, 2014: 154). Therefore we feel it is essential that all perioperative practitioners recognise the risks to compassionate care within the perioperative environment, so that they can take measures to mitigate against this, and to ensure that they promote the vision and values for good care, such as those expressed in the form of the 'six Cs' (Department of Health, 2012) and those recently highlighted values of being open and honest when things go wrong (HCPC, 2015). This text therefore has a clear focus on the patient as a person, and will illustrate the importance of caring for both a patient's physical and psychological needs in the perioperative setting.

Surgical intervention is considered to be the core component of perioperative care as this often directs all the other interventions and hence the perioperative plan of care;

for example, the type of surgical access required will directly influence patient positioning and the most appropriate type of anaesthesia. Equally important in our view, however, is consideration of the wider implications related to surgery and the perioperative
experience – for example, the long-term recovery implications and the impact upon the
patient, the quality of their life and indeed their lifestyle. We believe this is essential to
enable the practitioner to empathise with the patient and to provide effective holistic
care.

THE PERIOPERATIVE CARE SETTING

A patient will receive care in a number of different settings as part of their perioperative
journey – for example, outpatient clinics and surgical wards. The surgical intervention,
however, will usually take place within the operating department, which comprises
anaesthetic rooms, operating theatres, a post-anaesthetic care unit (PACU) and various
supporting services; and the care within these specific areas will be the core of this
text. However, no aspect of the perioperative journey can be considered in isolation as
each element directly impacts upon another, as is particularly evident in day surgery,
where a streamlined patient pathway is essential in order to facilitate the timely discharge of the patient.

The increase in day surgery is one of the most significant changes to perioperative
care as this is now considered 'the norm for elective surgery' (NHS Institute for Innovation and Improvement, 2008); this approach to surgery increases efficiency through
the release of inpatient beds and also improves patient experience. This investment in
day case surgery is largely due to two key changes, one related to the selection of
patients, the other to expansion of the infrastructure and service. Patient selection for
day surgery has developed to consider the patient's overall health rather than being
constrained by specific physiological boundaries – for example, American Society of
Anesthesiologists (ASA) status or body mass index (BMI). Consequently, the majority
of patients are considered suitable for day surgery unless there is a specific rationale
for an inpatient stay – for example, the anticipated postoperative pain is greater than
can be managed by oral analgesics (Verma *et al.*, 2011). The range of procedures performed in the day surgery setting has increased to include more complex surgical
interventions – for example, awake craniotomy and endovascular aneurysm stents; this
transition requires a review of the procedure to identify modifications that will enable
the patient to be discharged on the day of surgery – for example, altered analgesic
management (Verma *et al.*, 2011). These changes have presented new challenges for
the perioperative team and hence it is through their own professional development that
they are able to continue to meet the care needs of changing patient groups.

PATIENT SAFETY WITHIN THE PERIOPERATIVE ENVIRONMENT

The Department of Health (DH) (2013) prioritises patient safety as the central component of high-quality care, and this is particularly pertinent in the perioperative environment, which we consider to be high risk in recognition of the number of high-impact

interventions performed as part of each patient's care (Abbott and Wordsworth, 2014). In addition to safety, quality care in the NHS should deliver a patient-centred experience and should also be effective (DH, 2008, 2013); this need for an effective service is imperative to meet the demand requirements and has been highlighted by national initiatives such as the productive operating theatre.

The high-risk nature of the perioperative environment has resulted in a number of processes and procedures that are designed to ensure patient safety and will be employed for all the case studies in this text; there are also some specific checks that may be required for individual procedures or patients. The generic daily checks include a functional check of the theatre environment, including the environmental controls and a check of all surgical and anaesthetic equipment, in accordance with manufacturers' instructions and any local policy. In addition to functional checking, more comprehensive testing is also performed as part of a maintenance and calibration programme to ensure that all equipment continues to function correctly. There are also checking processes related directly to the care of the patient – for example, the World Health Organization (WHO) Surgical Safety Checklist, which is completed for all patients and explored later in this chapter. In addition, there are also intervention-specific checks – for example, those required when administering blood and blood products. All these procedures are designed to ensure the safe care of the patient in the operating department; however, technical errors are not the greatest threat to safety, rather it is human factors that present the greatest risk (Reason, 1995, 2005).

Human factors are particularly pertinent to the perioperative environment and this area can be defined as a scientific discipline that 'encompass[es] all those factors that can influence people and their behaviour. In a work context, human factors are the environmental, organisational and job factors, and individual characteristics which influence behaviour at work' (Clinical Human Factors Group, n.d.). Consequently it is important that all members of the perioperative team are able to recognise the non-technical factors that may impact upon the care of the patient – which may include fatigue, stress, poor team working and pressurised situations – and to manage these effectively to maintain quality of care.

THE MULTIDISCIPLINARY PERIOPERATIVE CARE TEAM

By acknowledging that the perioperative patient is cared for by a number of different practitioners during their perioperative journey we have designed this text to demonstrate the importance of effective communication by these professionals to ensure continuity of care. Within the operating department a multidisciplinary team (MDT) will care for the patient and in this section we will consider who makes up this team; this will include those directly employed by the operating department, medics employed by medical directorates in the hospital and practitioners from other departments when required for specific cases – for example, diagnostic radiographers for some trauma and urology cases.

The non-medical operating department team is a diverse team of a number of different practitioners undertaking different roles, and therefore it is important to understand the roles they will have in delivering care within the operating department. Registered practitioners within the operating department are generally employed under the generic role of 'theatre practitioner' or 'perioperative practitioner', and will practise in the anaesthetic care, surgical care and/or PACU (often called 'recovery'). This 'theatre/perioperative practitioner' workforce will comprise operating department practitioners (ODPs) and theatre nurses, and while a generic title is frequently employed to show parity in the roles, this is not the case at the point of registration. ODPs undertake pre-registration education specific to the care of the perioperative patient and as such have met the threshold standard for protection of the public: the Health and Care Professions Council (HCPC) Standards of Proficiency (HCPC, 2014). Unlike ODPs, nurses undertake generalist pre-registration education and may not necessarily visit the operating department as part of this programme; consequently they must undertake additional post-registration education to enable them to practise within the operating department. The National Safety Standards for Invasive Procedures (NatSSIPs) requirements related to staffing state that there must be 'an appropriate ratio holding a specific primary or postgraduate practice qualification applicable to the procedural area' (NHS England, 2015: 26) and the College of Operating Department Practitioners has advised that a minimum of one member of the non-medical surgical team must hold a specific qualification in perioperative care (CODP, 2015), thus demonstrating the importance of theatre nurses undertaking appropriate post-registration education. We have already highlighted that ODPs are the only professional group to undertake a nationally recognised pre-registration qualification specific to perioperative care (Abbott and Wordsworth, 2014) and for this reason this text will refer to the ODP role when discussing the input of the non-medical registrant workforce in the operating theatre, although it is acknowledged that, in some cases, this care may be delivered by an appropriately educated and trained nurse.

The operating department has a number of roles undertaken by healthcare support workers; within the UK, these staff members are currently not registered and therefore the primary responsibility for them lies with the employer; however there is ongoing debate regarding the most appropriate form of regulation for support workers (Lovegrove et al., 2013). There are a number of different healthcare support worker roles and these vary between operating departments throughout the UK; this is reflected in a range of local titles. This text uses the term 'perioperative support worker (PSW)' consistently to refer to a non-registered support worker within the operating department. These PSWs undertake a range of duties, which include circulating in theatre, supporting patients and staff in the PACU, collecting patients, and preparing the theatre for surgery. Some PSWs will undertake further education to become assistant theatre practitioners (ATPs), an intermediate role between that of a PSW and a registered member of staff. The ATP in the operating theatre will scrub for a defined list of cases, however this is under the delegation of a registrant who is present throughout the case and must perform the count of all accountable items (swabs, needles and instruments) with the ATP in addition to ensuring all documentation is completed correctly (PCC, 2015).

There are also a number of advanced non-medical roles within the operating department, however the adoption of these roles varies locally and therefore these practitioners will not be necessarily be present in all cases or hospitals. The surgical first assistant (SFA) is a registrant who provides continuous surgical assistance under the direct supervision of the operating surgeon; they do not undertake surgical intervention but undertake skills such as cutting of deep sutures, nerve and deep tissue retraction (retractors are placed by the surgeon), assisting with haemostasis (including indirect diathermy), suction and camera manipulation for endoscopic surgery (PCC, 2012). It is important to note that the SFA is an additional member of the surgical team; the scrub practitioner should not be working in a dual role and assuming SFA duties in addition to their scrub role for the specific case unless the individual hospital has a policy to support this practice (PCC, 2012). The Surgical Care Practitioner (SCP) and Physicians' Assistant (Anaesthesia) (PA(A)) are both advanced roles at postgraduate level, developed to meet the shortage of junior medics, and hence these practitioners will undertake the some elements of the medical role under the direction and supervision of a surgeon or anaesthetist (AAGBI, 2011; RCS, 2014).

In order to deliver safe, effective perioperative care, it is essential that the members of the MDT work together effectively and the case studies in this text demonstrate how effective team working is essential for continuity of care throughout the perioperative journey. All practitioners caring for the patient during the perioperative journey have a responsibility to promote continuity of care, and Abbott and Booth (2014) believe that this is reliant on the effective communication skills of the practitioners; consequently, record keeping is essential in all of the case studies. The interpersonal skills of the MDT members are also essential in contributing to an effective team as the different professional knowledge and philosophy of care will result in a range of important perspectives, and it is important therefore that these views are discussed in order to deliver the best possible care for the patient. In addition to the importance of communicating within the MDT, the team must also communicate effectively with the patient throughout the patient's experience, and it is this effective communication that allows the team to identify and respond to the patient's individual needs.

PROFESSIONAL, ETHICAL AND LEGAL ASPECTS OF PERIOPERATIVE CARE

There are a number of professional, ethical and legal aspects of perioperative care, and while these are often considered as a collective, it is important to note that, although there are some common elements, these are three distinct areas. When considering the responsibility of the practitioner with regard to these requirements, it is common to use the terms 'accountability' and 'responsibility', however these cannot be used interchangeably and it is important to note the distinct difference. Accountability can be defined as 'how far practitioners can be held to account for their actions or omissions' (Wordsworth, 2007: 192), hence accountability may be explored as part of legal proceedings or in the context of regulatory codes of conduct, and a practitioner must be able to justify their actions and decision making. By contrast, Wordsworth (2007: 192) states that 'responsibility places much more emphasis on task, role and action as opposed to decision-making'.

Working in accordance with the legal frameworks that direct perioperative care is essential for all members of the MDT and, as Booth (2014a: 83) asserts, 'there is no excuse for ignorance with regard to adhering to the legal requirements related to the ODP role'. There are many legal statutes that govern perioperative care – for example, the Health and Safety at Work Act 1973, the Equality Act 2010, the Public Interest

Disclosure Act 1998 and the Misuse of Drugs Act 1968 – however, there are many more legal statutes that will be considered appropriate in individual cases. All of the patient case studies in this text, however, will have given valid consent for their interventions, and although there is no English statute that defines the principles of consent, it has been established through case law that touching a patient without consent may be deemed the offence of battery (Booth, 2014a). Valid consent is given 'voluntarily by an informed person who has the capacity to consent to the intervention in question' (DH, 2009) and so the case studies in this text will explore any challenges related to obtaining consent if relevant to the given patient.

Practitioners who care for the patient within the perioperative setting are expected to deliver care in a professional manner, and this applies equally to all members of the team. Professionalism is considered 'a set of characteristics and qualities that transcend professional status and hierarchy' (Wordsworth, 2014: 162) and, consequently, the case studies in this text will demonstrate some of the different values and behaviours that are commensurate with professional behaviour. Registrant practitioners are accountable to their regulatory bodies for their professional behaviour and adherence to legal frameworks and standards of competence (Wordsworth, 2014); it is, however, important to clarify that an expectation to behave in a professional manner is not confined to those practitioners who have statutory registration or are part of a recognised profession.

Perioperative practitioners also need to have an appreciation of ethical principles, as they will encounter a number of ethical issues within their practice. These issues may also have a legal and professional component, however it should be noted that 'ethics' refers to 'a principle that guides human behaviour' and is therefore different from morals, which are 'associated with those that guide social behaviour' (Booth, 2014b: 98). There are a number of different ethical theories that enable perioperative practitioners to explore the ethical considerations of a particular issue, and some of these may be explored in the context of the case studies presented.

PATIENT ASSESSMENT IN THE PERIOPERATIVE CARE ENVIRONMENT

Having outlined the inherent complexity of the perioperative environment, it will come as little surprise to suggest that patient assessment and the role that ODPs play can also be naturally complex. Given that different professional groups share the occupational space, over time nurses and ODPs, together with the medical team (anaesthetic and surgical), have come to share overall responsibility for the assessment, planning and delivery of patient care.

Assessment of the operative list

As Abbott (2014: 189) has previously explored, it is usual for different professionals to undertake different assessments. These assessments are vitally important aspects of any surgery and anaesthetic intervention, and must be communicated effectively to enable the adaptation and optimisation of patient outcomes throughout all stages of the perioperative journey. Therefore patient safety initiatives such as the WHO Surgical Safety Checklist (2009) are inherent features of all the case studies that follow. We have taken the approach that these need not be replicated in each case study, but acknowledge that the checklist process will have been carried out in all cases in order to mitigate against patient harm caused through a range of factors, such as surgical infection, untoward anaesthetic incidents, and poor communication and team-working deficiencies. In all cases a three-phase approach includes:

1 sign in (takes place before induction of anaesthesia)
2 time out (takes place before surgery commences)
3 sign out (takes place at the point of wound closure and before transfer to the post-anaesthetic care unit).

However, it is also not unusual for the checklist to be adapted to meet localised needs, and it is thus included in local documentation. Where this is the case, and there is some deviation from the checklist as a result of the context of the patient care case study, then these particular adaptations will be explored. The five-step 'patient safety first' initiative, as a key feature of optimising effective team working and team culture, will also have taken place (NPSA, 2010) as an essential feature of patient assessment, which in addition to the Surgical Safety Checklist, includes an initial preoperative briefing to all of the team before the start of the list, and a final postoperative briefing stage designed to assess the effectiveness of the list, as well as to identify areas for improvement. It is important to be aware that these pre- and post- list briefings will be effective only if the whole team engage with them and remain in the theatre for the duration of the operating list; consequently it is essential that the team pause and perform another briefing whenever there are changes to the planned list, and that a full handover is performed whenever the team changes (NHS England, 2015).

Patient assessment and the perioperative journey

Due to our focus on the totality of patient care, each one of the case studies will acknowledge the importance of patient assessment throughout the perioperative journey. This includes aspects of preoperative preparation, admission, anaesthetic assessment, intraoperative assessment, post-anaesthetic assessment and discharge from the PACU. However, rather than simply list each one of these phases, our approach is to concentrate on aspects of assessment that are particularly important or relevant as a consequence of the context of the patient's condition and care needs, the type and complexity of the surgical and anaesthetic intervention, or a combination of these factors.

The case studies are not therefore intended to be prescriptive but demonstrate specific features and adaptations to patient care based on the individual patient's requirements. For example, each case study includes specific information on the preoperative preparation both prior to admission and at the point of admission. As Abbott (2014: 172) points out, this is because preoperative assessment is usually informed by local policy and specific screening tools 'that enable healthcare professionals to assess the patient and identify specific preoperative investigations or preparations that may be needed'. Importantly, these screening tools are needed to identify case complexity and any further detailed investigations including collaboration from other specialist services and health professionals. Where this is the case it will be explored in greater detail as a feature of the case study.

PREOPERATIVE ASSESSMENT

Similarly we take the view that all patients will have been exposed to detailed preoperative assessment, including past medical history, details of previous surgery and anaesthesia, baseline observations and any current medication. Assessment of the likelihood of venous thromboembolism (VTE) is also routinely undertaken and risk assessed according to NICE (2010) guidelines. This is because all perioperative patients, at some stage in their journey, will be immobile, and therefore they all have the VTE risk factor of venous stasis. As a consequence patients are ordinarily fitted with anti-embolism stockings and intermittent pneumatic pressure devices are often applied to the patient in the theatre, along with the possible use of pharmacological VTE prophylaxis. During admission all patients are routinely subjected to baseline observations, in addition to specific assessments such as the likelihood of requiring specific pressure area care.

Anaesthetic assessment

Anaesthetic assessment is a critical feature of any patient perioperative assessment and includes the essential features listed in the box.

Essential features of anaesthetic assessment

- Confirm patient's identity
- Review existing case notes
- Interview patient regarding past medical and anaesthetic history
- Undertake a physical examination, including airway assessment
- Review results of preoperative investigations
- Discuss with the patient the likely anaesthetic technique
- Explain preoperative fasting, pain relief and risks
- Confirm patient's understanding and obtain consent
- Record discussions in the anaesthetic record
- Prescribe pre-medication if required

Source: Adapted from RCoA (2009)

Again, where any of these present particular features of the patient's care, they are described in more detail – for example, where assessment has indicated the possibility of a difficult airway that requires a different technique, including the availability of specific and specialised equipment. Detailed history taking may also provide vital information, such as history of reflux, or even the existence of hereditary conditions that reveal the possibility of life-threatening conditions, such as malignant hyperthermia. Likewise an assessment of past medication history could have a particular relevance to the case study, such as the likelihood of interaction with existing medication with anaesthetic agents, or the implications of withdrawal of medication, as well as drug (or other) allergies.

Assessment at induction

When the patient is received in the operating theatre, usually by the ODP, a number of standardised checks are carried out, and it is important that patient identity and consent are confirmed. At this point the ODP should initiate a check for any allergies, and confirm the time when the patient last ate or drank. To enable this dialogue, the ODP should assess whether the patient requires any support such as hearing aids or glasses to help them read and communicate their consent. Explanation and consent should also be obtained for a number of baseline interventions such as non-invasive blood pressure (NIBP), electrocardiography (ECG), and importantly oxygen saturation via a pulse oximeter with verbal confirmation of correct placement and functionality, before induction is commenced (WHO, 2009). The NICE (2008) guidelines also recommend that the patient's temperature be taken prior to induction, preferably with a temporal scanner, which is considered more accurate than a tympanic thermometer.

In addition to any physical assessment the ODP has a vital role to play in assessing the patient's underlying emotional state, which is subject to heightened stress prior to and during anaesthesia and surgery. Because of this the case studies explore the individual support that each patient requires throughout their perioperative journey.

INTRAOPERATIVE PATIENT ASSESSMENT

Ongoing physiological device-based monitoring (NIBP, ECG, oxygen saturation) should continue during the intraoperative phase, and importantly the Association of Anaesthetists of Great Britain and Ireland (AAGBI, 2007) stipulates that these should be supported by further clinical assessment such as pulse palpation, pupil dilation, auscultation of breath sounds, chest and/or movement of a reservoir bag. Where muscle relaxants are deployed as part of the anaesthetic technique, a nerve stimulator must be available; and airway gases and resultant pressures, along with the patient's temperature, should also be recorded – the latter every 30 minutes (NICE, 2008). Further additional invasive monitoring in the form of arterial blood pressure and central venous pressure (CVP) may also feature and is explored further within the abdominal aortic aneurysm case study (Case Study 14).

In order to avoid the risk of awareness during general anaesthesia, an assessment of consciousness is also routinely carried out. Although a number of methods have been described to signpost the presence of light anaesthesia, the PRST score (see below) has been widely advocated. The criteria are individually awarded a score between 0 and 2, and the sum of these represents the degree of autonomic reflexive activity, and therefore the likely depth of anaesthesia (AnaesthesiaUK, 2005):

P (systolic blood pressure)
R (heart rate)
S (sweating)
T (tears).

Where appropriate, neuromuscular blockade is also routinely assessed through observation, typically through facial movements or muscle tone around the surgical site. The degree of blockade can also be calculated with the use of a peripheral nerve stimulator.

Each case study also assumes that effective fluid management has been deployed in order to maximise the patient's postoperative outcome. As such the ODP has a vital role to play in accurately monitoring fluid balance, which usually encompasses the calculation of blood loss from the operative site. This involves calculating blood volume in the suction bottle along with the volume of any irrigation fluid, which should be recorded accurately before being subtracted from the total volume of suctioned fluids. In many instances, blood loss would normally be calculated by weighing wet swabs before subtracting the dry swab weight.

POST-ANAESTHETIC CARE ASSESSMENT UNIT (PACU)

Along with highlighting the anaesthetic and surgical phases of the perioperative journey, the choice of case studies is also designed to highlight the contribution that the qualified recovery practitioner makes to the care of the patient. Starting with a handover from the anaesthetist, this should contain details of the care of the patient thus far, along with any specific recommendations in the immediate postoperative period. Again NIBP monitoring and pulse oximetry must be available, along with the capacity to undertake ECG, capnography and nerve stimulation (AAGBI, 2007). It is also anticipated that the patient's temperature will be recorded every 15 minutes, as per NICE (2008) guidelines.

Throughout the range of case studies it is important to note that the patient will arrive in the PACU in various stages of consciousness and the recovery practitioner is responsible for making a subsequent assessment of this. One-to-one care is advocated and regular assessment is required using the Airway, Breathing, Circulation, Disability, Exposure (ABCDE) algorithm, whereby specific features of the deployment of this algorithm and the care given are explored individually.

The assessment of pain is also a vital feature of postoperative care, and Abbott (2014) has suggested that the simplicity of the verbal rating scale makes it suitable in the early stages of recovery. The assessment of pain is however explored throughout the case studies using a range of assessment tools that are appropriate for the age and ability of the patient. Postoperative nausea and vomiting (PONV) is a complication that can delay patient recovery and therefore is assessed routinely in the PACU. This can be achieved using a number of verbal descriptive scales (VDS) or visual analogue scales, depending upon local policy and the appropriateness and abilities of the patients described in the case studies. The selected case studies will also explore the details of the application of AAGBI (2002) discharge criteria, which is again embedded within local protocols and procedures. Finally, in some of the case studies the recovery of the patient is described not just in relation to the immediate and short-term postoperative period, but also the medium- and, in some cases, longer-term recovery of the patient.

SUMMARY

This introduction has illustrated the complex nature of perioperative care, and the relationships between the patient and the wider perioperative environment, including the perioperative team, context and culture, in addition to the technical requirements of the many interventions performed as part of care delivery. The Department of Health (DH, 2013: 14) has stated that, 'the quality of patient care should come before all other considerations in the leadership and conduct of the NHS, and patient safety is the keystone dimension of quality'. Consequently all the case studies will encourage you to explore how care is delivered safely for the given patient. In support of the wider concept of patient experience, it is essential that the ODP understand the many facets of care delivery for the perioperative patient and can assimilate these to develop an individualised plan of care for each patient; hence these case studies will support the development of this important aspect of practice.

REFERENCES AND FURTHER READING

Abbott, H. (2014) Perioperative assessment, in Abbott, H., Ranson, M. and Braithwaite, W. (eds) *Clinical Examination Skills for Healthcare Professionals*. Keswick: M&K Publishing.

Abbott, H. and Booth, H. (2014) Working in the perioperative team, in Abbott, H. and Booth, H. (eds) *Foundations for Operating Department Practice*. Maidenhead: Open University Press.

Abbott, H. and Wordsworth, S. (2014) Improving safety culture: a profession in the fast lane. *Journal of Operating Department Practitioners*, **2**(6): 231–235.

AnaesthesiaUK (2005) Clinical signs. Available online at: www.frca.co.uk/article.aspx?articleid=100494 (accessed 30 October 2015).

Association of Anaesthetists of Great Britain and Ireland (AAGBI) (2002) *Immediate Postanaesthetic Recovery*. London: AAGBI.

Association of Anaesthetists of Great Britain and Ireland (AAGBI) (2007) *Recommendations for Standards of Monitoring During Anaesthesia and Recovery* (4th edn). London: AAGBI.

Association of Anaesthetists of Great Britain and Ireland (AAGBI) (2011) *Physicians' Assistants (Anaesthesia) Review 2011*. London: AAGBI.

Booth, H. (2014a) Legal frameworks for operating department practitioners, in Abbott, H. and Booth, H. (eds) *Foundations for Operating Department Practice*. Maidenhead: Open University Press.

Booth, H. (2014b) Ethics for the operating department practitioner, in Abbott, H. and Booth, H. (eds) *Foundations for Operating Department Practice*. Maidenhead: Open University Press.

Clinical Human Factors Group (n.d.) What is human factors? Available online at: http://chfg.org/what-is-human-factors (accessed 27 October 2015).

College of Operating Department Practitioners (CODP) (2015) Guidance on local implementation of the NHS England National Safety Standards for Invasive Procedures (NatSSIPs) – Workforce Issues. Available online at: www.unison.org.uk/content/uploads/2014/07/CODP_NatSSIPS_Position_Statement.pdf (accessed 27 October 2015).

Council of Deans of Health (2013) ODP pre-registration programmes educational threshold; Council of Deans of Health position statement October 2013. Available online at: www.councilofdeans.org.uk/wp-content/uploads/2013/10/ODP-BSc-Threshold-position-20131030-final1.pdf (accessed 31 October 2013).

Department of Health (DH) (2008) High quality care for all: NHS next stage review final report. Available online at: www.gov.uk/government/uploads/system/uploads/attachment_data/file/228836/7432.pdf (accessed 24 February 2014).

Department of Health (DH) (2009) *Reference Guide to Consent for Examination or Treatment*. London: Department of Health.

Department of Health (DH) (2012) Compassion in practice. Available online at: www.england.nhs.uk (accessed 3 February 2016).

Department of Health (DH) (2013) A promise to learn – a commitment to act: improving the safety of patients in England. Available online at: www.gov.uk/government/uploads/system/uploads/attachment_data/file/226703/Berwick_Report.pdf (accessed 1 September 2013).

Health and Care Professions Council (HCPC) (2014) *Standards of Proficiency, Operating Department Practitioners*. London: Health and Care Professions Council.

Health and Care Professions Council (HCPC) (2015) Duty of candour – PSA progress report. Executive summary and recommendations. Available online at: www.hcpc-uk.org/assets/documents/10004A67Enc03-Dutyofcandour-PSAprogressreport.pdf (accessed 30/10/2015).

Lovegrove, M., Jelfs, E., Wheeler, I. and Davis, J. (2013) *The Higher Education Contribution to Education and Training for Healthcare Support Worker Roles*. London: Council of Deans of Health and Skills for Health.

National Institute for Health and Clinical Excellence (NICE) (2008) Inadvertent perioperative hypothermia. *NICE Clinical Guideline 65*. London: National Institute for Health and Clinical Excellence.

National Institute for Health and Clinical Excellence (NICE) (2010) *Venous Thromboembolism: Reducing the Risk*. London: National Institute for Health and Clinical Excellence.

National Patient Safety Agency (NPSA) (2010) *Five Steps to Safer Surgery*. London: National Patient Safety Agency.

NHS Confederation (2014) Key statistics on the NHS. Available online at: www.nhsconfed.org/resources/key-statistics-on-the-nhs (accessed 22 August 2014).

NHS England (2015) National Safety Standards for Invasive Procedures (NatSSIPs). Available online at: www.england.nhs.uk/patientsafety/never-events/natssips/ (accessed 27 October 2015).

NHS Institute for Innovation and Improvement (2008) Treat day surgery as the norm. Available online at: www.institute.nhs.uk/quality_and_service_improvement_tools/quality_and_service_improvement_tools/day_surgery_-_treat_day_surgery_as_the_norm.html (accessed 29 January 2012).

Perioperative Care Collaborative (PCC) (2012) Position statement: surgical first assistant, Perioperative Care Collaborative. Available online at: www.afpp.org.uk (accessed 27 October 2015).

Perioperative Care Collaborative (PCC) (2015) Optimising the contribution of the perioperative support worker. Available online at: www.afpp.org.uk (accessed 27 October 2015).

Reason, J. (1995) Understanding adverse events: human factors. *Quality in Health Care*, **4**: 80–89.

Reason, J. (2005) Safety in the operating theatre. Part 2: Human error and organisational failure. *Quality and Safety in Health Care*, **1**: 56–61.

Royal College of Anaesthetists (RCoA) (2009) Guidance on the provision of anaesthesia services for pre-operative care, in RCoA (ed.) *Guidelines for the Provision of Anaesthetic Services* (rev. edn). London: Royal College of Anaesthetists.

Royal College of Surgeons (RCS) (2014) *The Curriculum Framework for the Surgical Care Practitioner*. London: Royal College of Surgeons.

Verma, R., Alladi, R., Jackson, I., Johnston, I., Kumar, C., Page, R., Smith, I., Stocker, M., Tickner, C., Williams, S. and Young, R. (2011) Day case and short stay surgery: 2. *Anaesthesia*, **66**: 417–434.

Woodhead, K. and Fudge, L. (2012) The context of perioperative care, in Woodhead, K. and Fudge, L. (eds) *Manual of Perioperative Care: An Essential Guide*. Chichester: John Wiley & Sons.

Wordsworth, S. (2007) Accountability in perioperative practice, in Smith, B., Rawling, P., Wicker, P. and Jones, C. (eds) *Core Topics in Operating Department Practice, Anaesthesia and Critical Care*. Cambridge: Cambridge University Press.

Wordsworth, S. (2014) Professional practice for operating department practitioners, in Abbott, H. and Booth, H. (eds) *Foundations for Operating Department Practice: Essential Theory for Practice*. Maidenhead: Open University Press.

World Health Organization (WHO) (2009) *Implementation Manual Surgical Safety Checklist* (2nd edn). Geneva: World Health Organization.

PART 1
Suggested 1st Year (Level 4) Case Studies

CASE STUDY 1

Circumcision: the care of Donald Driscoll

Romilly Norman

INTRODUCTION AND LEARNING OUTCOMES

A circumcision procedure is a minor urological operation; it takes on average 20 minutes of surgical time, and the majority of cases are performed under a general anaesthetic (GA). However, this case study will demonstrate to the reader that the patient had pre-existing co-morbidities that required additional pre-assessment investigations, resulting in a change to the standard anaesthetic plan.

By the end of this case study you will be able to:

- describe the surgical technique used to carry out an adult circumcision
- explain how the patient receives individual perioperative care, and how this is adapted to the patient's requirements
- understand the complete surgical journey of an adult patient undergoing a circumcision, gaining an appreciation of the role of the multidisciplinary team (MDT).

Case outline

Donald Driscoll was a 75-year-old white Irish widower who lived alone in his own house situated on the outskirts of the town. The retired mechanic had two children; only his daughter lives locally, with her husband and three children. Donald and his daughter do not see each other regularly, yet he does have a small support network in the form of neighbours and two close friends. Donald presented to his GP with tightening and irritation of the foreskin and glans. On closer inspection by the GP, he identified the external urethral opening had decreased in size; however, the patient was not in urinary retention. Donald proceeded to mention that he had first noticed the changes three months prior to this appointment.

---

1 How would the GP arrive at a diagnosis?

A An examination was carried out and the GP asked Donald to describe his symptoms in detail. The patient described the daily inconvenience of having to cope with the

3

irritation and soreness around the 'tip' of his penis. Donald had not immediately sought any medical advice as he put his condition down to the effects of ageing. Over recent weeks, the initial irritation had progressed to pain and swelling. In addition to physical assessment a urine sample was taken, plus a blood test to determine the patient's glucose level, to eliminate diabetes, along with a microbial swab to rule out any infection. Donald returned to his GP three weeks later for a follow-up appointment to find that the tests for infection and diabetes had shown negative results and his glucose level was within the normal limits of 4.0–5.9 mmol/L.

2 **Could you describe Donald's initial care?**

A The GP was able to diagnose chronic balanitis, which is a long-term yet treatable condition. Balanitis is swelling of the foreskin or the head of the penis and a non-retractile foreskin (Malone and Steinbrecher, 2007). The GP instructed Donald to clean his genital area, particularly under and around the foreskin, to reduce the irritation and to prevent infection. The patient was advised to wash regularly with non-perfumed products to rule out the possibility that the irritation was caused by an allergic reaction. An urgent referral to a specialist urology team was not considered necessary but, after waiting ten weeks, Donald was assessed by the senior registrar. As the condition was unlikely to improve, and given Donald's age and ability to monitor his genital area carefully, a circumcision procedure was considered to be the best option. Donald was happy to accept that this was his best option and was keen for the procedure to be undertaken as soon as possible.

> ### Stop and think
>
> What do you think are the main advantages of a pre-assessment clinic?
>
> Two weeks prior to the operation date Donald attended a pre-assessment clinic to allow the medical and nursing team to prepare and optimise his surgical care. The registered nurse (RN) commenced the integrated care plan (ICP) used to record Donald's care at different stages of the patient's journey provided by the multidisciplinary team (MDT). The nurse took a full holistic and medical history, including baseline observations (BP, heart rate, SpO_2, weight and height). A member of the anaesthetic and surgical team also reviewed Donald, and the anaesthetist in particular became aware of a number of co-morbidities that they felt it was important to consider.

3 **What is meant by co-morbidities and how might they affect Donald?**

A Co-morbidities are two or more chronic illnesses/diseases that run concurrently or sequentially, requiring more complex clinical management.

   Donald was being treated for hypertension (high blood pressure), which can be the cause and effect of conditions such as chronic heart failure (Page and McKinney, 2012). Donald had been prescribed ramipril, which works by reducing the production of angiotensin II, widening the blood vessels. This improves blood flow around the body, as well as ensuring that the heart pumps more efficiently. Hence, this reduces blood pressure to within the normal parameters.

Although Donald had smoked heavily for most of his adult life, prior to giving up he had reduced the number to five to ten cigarettes per day. Because of his long-term addiction to nicotine he had been diagnosed with the emphysema that had manifested as chronic obstructive pulmonary disease (COPD). COPD is an uncompromising and non-reversible condition in which, over time, the airway becomes narrowed due to damage to the alveoli as well as loss of lung elasticity (GOLD, 2011). The symptoms of the disease are fatigue, persistent cough with phlegm, and breathlessness (dyspnoea), which worsens over time but can manifest as an acute exacerbation (NICE, 2010). Donald takes a prescribed daily dose of bronchodilators in conjunction with a steroid, and Ventolin inhaler. Because of his high risk of chest infections, he has had the influenza vaccine and has not had a hospital admission because of this condition. He does get breathless when walking on level ground, on average at ten minutes.

4 **Can you reflect on how these particular co-morbidities might impact on the patient's perioperative care?**

A The anaesthetic team were particularly concerned in terms of the patient's suitability for a GA, as anaesthesia can have a negative impact on hypertension and COPD. Due to inflammation of the airways, the expiratory airflow is limited, which impacts the patency of the small airways, and hence can affect both ventilation and perfusion. If severe cases of COPD are not managed appropriately, they can lead to respiratory failure (Lumb and Biercamp, 2013).

To be able to assess Donald's suitability for surgery and anaesthesia, a full blood count (FBC), urea and electrolytes (U&Es) were requested to ascertain kidney function, as well as an ECG based on the patient's age and hypertension. Finally, as a result of his COPD, Donald underwent a lung function test to ascertain his lung capacity. He was able to use the drop-in service at the lung function clinic on the same day as his pre-assessment appointment. This involved a spirometry test to identify the amount of exhaled air from one breath after a deep intake of breath, known as forced vital capacity (FVC). The second part of the test established the forced expiratory volume (FEV), measured at 1 second (FEV1) to provide an indication of airflow obstruction. The tests also provided data on total lung capacity (TLC) at the point of inhaling, and the functional residual capacity (FRC), which measured air in the lungs after exhaling (Loveridge, 2013). Based on a full medical history, physical examination and the lung function tests, Donald was found to have significantly reduced lung capacity and evidence of airflow obstruction, which, although improved after bronchodilators, was felt not to be suitable for a GA.

He had two choices: a spinal (regional anaesthesia) or a penile block under local anaesthetic (LA). The doctor explained all aspects of both anaesthetics as well as providing reading material, enabling Donald to make an informed choice in his own time.

Stop and think

Consider how both clinical guidelines and clinical decision making are used to devise and adapt patient care.

Initially, when seen in the pre-assessment clinic, the anaesthetist, guided by the NICE (2003a) Clinical Guidelines, ascertained that Donald's American Society of Anaesthesiologists (ASA) score was Grade 3, representing mild systemic disease. According to the guidelines, this suggested that further testing was not necessary (NICE, 2003b). However, because of Donald's existing co-morbidities, the anaesthetist was sufficiently concerned to investigate the patient's condition further. In the perioperative setting, the practitioner should be aware that what may appear to be routine surgery can be complicated by unexpected surgical difficulty. The patient's suitability for surgery or anaesthesia can often depend upon a range of factors, in particular the patient's physiological condition and the risks associated with any intervention.

5   **How was Donald prepared preoperatively?**

A   Donald's ICP was continued from pre-assessment, his baseline observations were taken on admission (BP 165/82, HR 90 bpm, SpO_2 94% on air, and temperature 36.6°C). Although the BP and heart rate were higher than average for this patient, it was possible that the unfamiliar surroundings and his anxiety over the operation were having an effect. Although Donald was not fit for a GA and was having a spinal anaesthetic, he was still required to be nil by mouth in case there should be a reason to convert to a GA in an emergency situation. Patients undergoing surgery with a spinal anaesthetic are also often sedated and this again could increase the likelihood of regurgitation and aspiration of stomach contents (Brady *et al.*, 2003). Donald was advised to continue to take his prescribed medication but with only a sip of water.

As well as being told of the benefits of a spinal anaesthetic, the anaesthetist also informed the patient about the associated complications, and the fact that if the spinal were to fail then the procedure would have to be performed under local anaesthesia in the form of a penile block.

> **Stop and think**
>
> Can you list the major complications associated with spinal anaesthesia in order of severity? The answers are given in Box 1.1.

Donald had an opportunity to put questions to the surgeon and, although he understood what was going to happen, he was concerned about how long it would be before he was able to drive. Given that he was about to undergo surgery this may seem trivial, however Donald is proud of his independence and sees his ability to continue to drive as a key feature of his independence. The surgeon advised him of the legal requirement that he could not drive until he was able to perform an emergency stop safely. For this reason he could not see a problem with him being able to drive after at least 24 hours, provided that there were no complications and he had recovered suitably from the spinal anaesthetic.

Having emphysema, hypertension and being over 60 put Donald at risk of venous thromboembolism (VTE). The surgeon assessed the risk and put the necessary

preventative measures in place, correctly measured knee-high compression stockings, and prescribed IV fluids until he could eat and drink.

Box 1.1: Complications associated with spinal anaesthesia, in order of severity

- Nerve damage
- Spinal haematoma
- Spinal infection
- Possible drug administration error
- Systemic toxicity
- Respiratory depression
- Hypotension
- Confusion in older people
- Pruritus/urinary retention/nausea
- Technical failure

Source: AnaesthesiaUK (2005)

---

6 **From the perspective of the operating department practitioner (ODP), how was the patient positioned in order to maximise the chance of a successful anaesthestic technique?**

A Donald was collected for theatre, and checks on the ward were carried out in relation to his name, date of birth, hospital number, any allergies, and when he last ate and drank. The consent form, anaesthetic chart and full notes were made available and accompanied Donald to the anaesthetic room. Donald was greeted by the anaesthe-tist and the ODP, and – following confirmation of identity checks and consent – routine monitoring was applied (non-invasive blood pressure, three-lead ECG and tempera-ture). An intravenous (IV) cannula was inserted into the less dominant hand, enabling venous access and at the same time allowing the patient to move around more eas-ily. A warmed one-litre bag of IV Hartmann's solution was titrated slowly to offset the risk of hypotension as a result of vasodilation following spinal anaesthetic. The World Health Organization (WHO) checklist was completed. The patient was then given the midazolam in order to reduce his anxiety.

Adopting the correct patient position can be critical to the success of the spinal anaesthetic technique as a whole, both in terms of identifying the correct anatomy and optimising the position to insert the spinal needle. The patient was manoeuvred on to the operating table then helped into a sitting position for the spinal, with his feet placed on a sturdy stool. He was asked to lower his arms and shoulders, and to place his chin on to his chest. He was given a pillow to hold on to around his abdo-men and then asked to push his back against the anaesthetist's fingers. This posi-tion opens up the spaces in between the spinal vertebrae to facilitate the insertion of the spinal needle. The spinal itself was performed by the anaesthetist, using an aseptic technique, with assistance from the ODP. They also carried out verbal and observational checks on the monitoring and with Donald, to guard against any untoward physiological response.

7 **Explain how a spinal anaesthetic would be undertaken.**

A At the site of the proposed introduction of the spinal needle the patient's skin was first numbed with 1% lidocaine, using a small-gauge needle to reduce discomfort. Due to the relatively short operating time, 2.5 ml of 0.5% Marcain Heavy® was prepared for the spinal; this would provide sufficient anaesthesia for surgery up to two hours. The ODP was able to help Donald remain as still as possible and gauge how well he was tolerating the insertion of the needle; the anaesthetist was then able to respond accordingly to any pain or discomfort. When the needle advanced through the dura mater into the subarachnoid space, a flashback of cerebrospinal fluid (CSF) was seen in the 25 gauge spinal needle, at which point the needle was confirmed as being in the right place and the Marcain Heavy® was administered. The drug takes an average five to eight minutes to take full effect, but the ODP informed the patient that he may also feel some immediate effects such as a 'warm and tingly' or 'heavy' feeling in his legs. A post-spinal BP was taken, with Donald now lying back down, and once a sufficient degree of block had been achieved to allow surgery, the surgical team were allowed to proceed.

8 **How was Donald cared for intraoperatively?**

A To ensure that, during the surgery, Donald's hands were kept away from the sterile field they were secured against his chest, while his elbows and heels were protected with gel padding to prevent pressure sore development or redness. On this occasion, due to the relatively short surgical time, intermittent pneumatic calf compressors were not required.

A screen was attached to the table at the level of the chest for two reasons: (1) to keep the large sterile drapes away from patient's face; (2) more importantly, so that Donald was not able to see the operation, which could potentially be very distressing. Once the surgical team were ready, the ODP sat with Donald during the entire procedure, holding his hand to provide reassurance and allowing him to speak when he chose to. Feeling anxious and fearful of the procedure and the unknown surroundings, Mitchell (2008) identified that patients need theatre staff throughout the procedure, not just for surgical reasons but for reassurance and to provide some normality. The ODP involved other members of the team with the conversation to help the patient relax, thereby reducing anxiety.

The anaesthetist recorded baseline observations on the anaesthetic chart and the patient's SpO_2 remained unchanged, therefore oxygen was not required. His BP remained constant and within normal limits and, therefore, remedial treatment of hypotension caused by the spinal was not required. Ephedrine 3 mg/ml was available to be administered every three to four minutes up to a maximum dose of 30 mg (British National Formulary (BNF), 2014). As an alternative, metaraminol 15–100 mg could also be used and additional fluids administered.

The scrub practitioner and the circulating practitioner performed the needle, swab and instrument count prior to allowing the surgeon to prepare the patient with Savlon. Before the surgeon and scrub practitioner prepped and draped, the ODP commenced with the second part of the WHO checklist, with all the team participating. Once the entire team was ready, the surgeon tested the spinal by pinching the foreskin lightly with toothed forceps, prior to commencement of surgery.

9   **Can you describe the surgical technique of an adult circumcision?**

A   The surgeon required only four different surgical instruments: a blade, four artery forceps, bipolar forceps and a needle holder. The artery forceps are clamped at 1 o'clock, 3 o'clock, 9 o'clock and 11 o'clock, all with equal tension. Once the blade cut around the marked area of the foreskin, bleeding occurred and haemostasis was achieved using bipolar forceps. Bipolar is an electrical current that runs from the machine to the forceps, which cauterises the vessel(s). The foreskin that had been removed was not sent as a histology specimen, which is normal procedure unless there was any reason for a tissue biopsy. The surgeon closed the edges of the wound using mattress stitch and a Vicryl Rapide suture. This is a braided suture that is easily knotted and has a strong tensile strength. This suture is also advantageous for the patient on two levels: first, the suture is soft and less likely to catch on clothing; second, as it is absorbable the patient does not need to attend his GP surgery or outpatients to have it removed.

After the surgical site had been cleaned with saline and then dried, a gauze dressing impregnated with paraffin (Jelonet) was applied to the wound. To keep the Jelonet dressing in place, and to act as a pressure dressing, the surgeon used blue non-raytec swabs with transpore tape. However, Molokwu and Peracha (2014) suggest using a condom over the dressing, which is adapted by cutting the top off to enable the patient to urinate normally. With the dressing in place, the ODP completed the 'sign out' component of the WHO checklist, and established that the full swab, needle and instrument count was correct.

10   **Consider which routine observations would have been made during the immediate postoperative period, and describe these.**

A   The handover to the staff in the PACU included information on the drugs used for the spinal anaesthetic, medical history and the postoperative plan of care. Sitting up in bed, Donald was able to breathe normally, however if his saturations decreased at any time, oxygen had been prescribed. The IV fluids were to be discontinued once the only bag of fluids had finished. The PACU practitioner's task was to ensure the patient was sent to the ward in a way that was comfortable and pain free, and that he was prepared for discharge. The patient's basic observations (BP, heart rate, respiration and SpO_2) continued to be monitored, as well as his temperature. This was expected to decrease, not because of the lower temperature in theatre but through some loss of body heat from the exposed area. This was corrected simply by applying blankets and bedding. The patient's observations were recorded following the Modified Early Warning Score (MEWS). MEWS is used widely on surgical patients, ensuring that any deterioration is recognised without delay and suitable management commenced. Scoring in such a systematic way gave clarity and provided an objective method of ascertaining when Donald was medically ready to be discharged from the PACU. By using the MEWS system, alongside monitoring of the wound, the patient stayed in the PACU for approximately one hour.

11 Can you describe what happened in terms of care for Donald back on the ward and up to his discharge from hospital?

A Donald's care was handed over to the ward nurse with a full discussion including the postop surgical instructions for the ward nurse and patient. Donald was discharged on the day of surgery once he had had something to eat and drink, and the spinal anaesthetic had completely worn off with additional pain relief available. Additionally, as one of the side effects of the spinal is urinary retention and due to the site of the surgery, Donald had to pass urine without concern.

Donald's discharge instructions were minimal. He was discharged not only from hospital on the day of surgery but also from the urology clinic, with no long-term future concerns of follow-up. For pain relief, he was recommended to use paracetamol available over the counter and advised not to get the area wet for 48 hours. Because the sutures were absorbable, he was not required to see the practice nurse, but was told how to identify the signs of infection and delayed healing. His final requirement was to have someone stay with him overnight in case of any postoperative complications; Donald had arranged for his daughter to stay with him.

REFERENCES AND FURTHER READING

AnaesthesiaUK (2005) Complications of regional anaesthesia. Available online at: www.frca.co.uk/article.aspx?articleid=100508 (accessed 8 September 2015).

Brady, M., Kinn, S., Stuart, P. and Ness, V. (2003) Preoperative fasting for adults to prevent perioperative complications. Available online at: http://onlinelibrary.wiley.com/doi/10.1002/14651858.CD004423/full (accessed 18 March 2014).

British National Formulary (BNF) (2014) Ephedrine hydrochloride, in Britain RPSoG (ed.) *The British National Formulary (BNF)*. London: BMJ Publishing Group.

Global Initiative for Chronic Obstructive Lung Disease (GOLD) (2011) Global strategy for the diagnosis, management, and prevention of chronic obstructive pulmonary disease. Available online at: www.goldcopd.org/guidelines-gold-summary-2011.html (accessed 8 September 2015).

Loveridge, C. (2013) Spirometry 3: interpreting the test. *Practice Nursing*, **24**(8): 382–386.

Lumb, A. and Biercamp, C. (2013) Chronic obstructive pulmonary disease and anaesthesia. *Continuing Education in Anaesthesia, Critical Care & Pain*, 30 May, pp. 1–5.

Malone, P. and Steinbrecher, H. (2007) Medical aspects of male circumcision. *British Medical Journal*, **335**: 1206–1209.

Mitchell, M. (2008) Conscious surgery: influence of the environment on patient anxiety. *Journal of Advanced Nursing*, **64**(3): 261–271.

Molokwu, C. and Peracha, A. (2014) Securing the dressing after circumcision in adults. *Annals of the Royal College of Surgeons*, **96**: 170.

National Institute for Clinical Excellence (NICE) (2003a) Grade 2 surgery (intermediate). Available online at: http://publications.nice.org.uk/preoperative-tests-cg3/guidance#grade-2-surgery-intermediate (accessed 12 March 2014).

National Institute for Clinical Excellence (NICE) (2003b) Preoperative tests: the use of routine preoperative tests for elective surgery. Available online at: www.nice.org.uk/guidance/cg3/chapter/guidance#grade-3-surgery-major (accessed 12 March 2014).

National Institute for Health and Clinical Excellence (NICE) (2010) Chronic obstructive pulmonary disease: management of chronic obstructive pulmonary disease in adults in primary and secondary care (partial update). Available online at: www.nice.org.uk/guidance/cg101 (accessed 8 September 2015).

Page, K. and McKinney, A. (2012) *Nursing the Acutely Ill Adult: Case Book.* Maidenhead: Open University Press.

Dynamic hip screw: the care of Enid Jones

Simon Nixon

INTRODUCTION AND LEARNING OUTCOMES

About 70,000–75,000 fractures of the hip occur each year, and this number is expected to increase year on year as the UK population ages (National Institute for Health and Clinical Excellence (NICE), 2011). This case study will enable readers to use an evidence-based approach (Aveyard and Sharp, 2013) to the management and treatment of an older adult who has sustained a fractured neck of femur as they go from point of injury to discharge from hospital. The primary focus of this case study is on the three phases of the perioperative environment: anaesthesia, surgery and post-anaesthetic care. This case study will emphasise the need for a multi-professional approach to deliver patient-centred care in order to maximise optimal patient outcomes.

By the end of this case study you will be able to:

- describe and explore the journey of an older adult patient who has had a fractured neck of femur surgically repaired using a dynamic hip screw
- discuss the role of the ODP in the care of the older adult orthopaedic patient
- optimise care for the older adult patient to ensure the best outcomes following surgical intervention.

Case outline

Enid Jones is an older adult, aged 81, who lives on her own in a small self-contained bungalow that is part of a warden-supported community. Despite her age she maintains her independence and enjoys the company of other residents, many of whom she has known for a number of years. Her husband died five years previously and she has a son and daughter, both of whom are married with families who live a distance from her. Enid's health is generally good, but she has been diagnosed as having a mild degree of osteoporosis, which was found during a local screening programme. This screening programme was initiated by Enid's local GP implementing the recommendations of the NICE (2012) *Clinical Guideline* 'Osteoporosis: assessing the risk of fragility fracture'.

Enid sustained her fracture after she fell while out shopping at her local supermarket. After she fell she was in a lot of pain and unable to stand unaided. She was assisted into a chair outside the supermarket by a number of concerned members of the public and staff from the supermarket, including one of its first aiders. An ambulance was called and efforts were made to make Enid as comfortable as possible while waiting for the paramedics to arrive. During this wait reassurance was given by the first aider and no fluids were given despite Enid's request for a cup of tea. Enid became a little agitated as the injury became more painful, and was concerned about her friends not being aware of where she was.

When the paramedics arrived they carried out a primary assessment followed by a secondary assessment (Fellows and Fellows, 2012); a preliminary diagnosis of a fracture of Enid's left hip was made on the basis of some shortening of the limb, pain over the injury site and patient history. It was decided to give morphine as an analgesic, make Enid as comfortable as possible and transport her to the local hospital, which had an orthopaedic service, as rapid surgical treatment reduces mortality and gives better outcomes (Egol and Strauss, 2009; NICE, 2011). Enid persuaded the paramedics to contact the warden at her place of residence and gave permission for the warden to inform her friends and next of kin.

1 **How would you ensure the preoperative optimisation of Enid's care?**

A Surgical fixation of the hip is considered to be the gold standard level of care because it allows early mobilisation and a reduced hospital stay, and this helps reduce co-morbidities such as deep vein thrombosis, pulmonary embolism, urinary tract and respiratory infections, and pressure ulcers (Egol and Strauss, 2009; White, Khan and Smitham, 2011). Enid was seen by a member of the orthopaedic team and an anaesthetist as soon as possible after her admission to the Emergency Department (ED) and, following examination and a series of tests, she was booked in for surgical fixation on her fractured hip later that day on the planned trauma list. The examination consisted of blood tests to check on anaemia, anticoagulation status and electrolyte balance, in addition to a check to establish whether Enid was a diabetic. Baseline vital signs were established: pulse, temperature, respiration and blood pressure data were all recorded. Physical tests were carried out to check that Enid did not have any acute or chronic chest or cardiac problems; these checks included electrocardiogram (ECG) and a chest x-ray, in addition to pelvis and lateral hip x-rays, as suggested by NICE *Clinical Guidelines* (2011). In addition to visits from the anaesthetist and surgeon, Enid was seen by the operating department practitioner (ODP), who would then continue her postoperative care in the post-anaesthetic care unit (PACU).

Enid was booked from the emergency department (ED) to the operating theatre to wait for an available slot on the trauma list. As Enid was nil by mouth at this point, an infusion of Hartmann's solution was started at this point, both to reduce the possibility of dehydration and to allow intravenous access for further pain relief if required.

This did mean, though, that she had to wait in a transit area within the ED, but she was assessed on a regular basis for pain and pressure area care.

Stop and think

What kinds of choices was Enid able to make about her own care plan and treatment?

A diagnosis of a non-displaced extracapsular left hip fracture was made, which required the insertion of a 'dynamic hip screw' (DHS) to relieve pain and restore mobility. DHS is considered to be the gold standard treatment for unstable but reduced neck of femur fractures (AO Foundation, 2014). Enid's treatment was discussed with her, and she was considered competent to make decisions about her care and able to consent for her surgery. The consideration of competence is considered fundamental in respecting the rights, in this case autonomy, of the patient (Melia, 2014). Enid was then offered a general anaesthetic (GA) or a spinal anaesthetic combined with a sedative. The implications of both techniques were discussed with her during her assessment by the anaesthetist. Enid was agreeable to the idea of a spinal anaesthetic because of her own and her friends' past experiences of postoperative nausea and vomiting (PONV). She was however made aware that there may be a requirement to change to GA for a number of reasons, and she agreed to this. Enid's nursing care and plan in the ED was based upon the ASPIRE model: Assess, Systematic nursing diagnosis, Plan, Implement, Re-check and Evaluate (Barrett, Wilson and Woollands, 2012). This care model is a continuous process, which ensured that Enid's basic care needs – including both her psychological and sociological needs – were met.

---

2 **With Enid in mind, can you describe the most appropriate anaesthetic technique and consider which drugs could be administered as part of her perioperative care?**

A It is important to note that routine preparation of the anaesthetic room had taken place at the beginning of the scheduled trauma list; this included checking of the anaesthetic machine by both the ODP and anaesthetist as per the manufacturer's guidelines and Association of Anaesthetists for Great Britain and Ireland (AAGBI) guidelines (AAGBI, 2012). After discussion with the anaesthetist, the ODP who was working in this area prepared the equipment that was anticipated to be required for Enid's surgery.

Anaesthetic technique and airway management

Enid had agreed to undergo a spinal anaesthetic, this being a subarachnoid block at the L3/L4 level, which is a sterile procedure that introduces a local anaesthetic solution into the cerebrospinal fluid (CSF). This is considered an alternative to general anaesthesia (GA) for patients with hip fractures, with the advantages that it is short acting, the anaesthetic effect lasting up to two hours, which promotes early mobilisation – a key issue in the care of elderly patients (Egol and Strauss, 2009; NICE, 2011). It also reduces PONV and avoids the issues associated with GA around respiratory depression (Hamlin, Richardson-Tench and Davies, 2009). In addition to spinal anaesthesia, Enid was given some sedation in the form of ketamine. Enid was expected to support her own airway, and oxygen would be available via a Hudson mask if required.

Pharmacological interventions and rationale

Ketamine was given to Enid to provide some sedation and to reduce the possibility of bronchospasm. It also enables a temporary dissociative anaesthetic state, providing some analgesia and amnesia, although it can cause postoperative nausea and vomiting and some visual hallucinations (Hatfield, 2014). A loading dose of ketamine was given as a bolus and then an infusion made up of 12 mg per kg per hour was used to maintain Enid's dissociative state.

Heavy bupivacaine was the local anaesthetic agent of choice for Enid's spinal anaesthesia (Allman and Wilson, 2011) as it can last up to two hours for good analgesic effect, but can provide up to four hours' postoperative pain relief.

To prevent infection, Enid was given 1 g of cefuroxime prophylactically during induction, which is considered best practice for all patients undergoing hip surgery (Egol and Strauss, 2009).

3   **What specific attention should be given to the patient's position in order to optimise Enid's surgery?**

A   Patient positioning is key to good surgical outcome (Hamlin *et al.*, 2009); it is about getting the balance right between surgical requirements, anaesthetic requirement and avoiding unnecessary harm to the patient. As Enid was considered an older adult, particular consideration was given to pressure ulcer prevention, DVT prevention and the possibility that some of Enid's joints were perhaps not as flexible as those of a younger patient. It was decided to position Enid supine, but with the fracture table attachments so access was available for x-ray imaging via the C-arm (image intensifier).

The positioning of Enid was supervised by the operating surgeon and the anaesthetist, and the ODPs made sure that the required padding, additional pillows, table attachments and warming blanket were all prepared in advance. Additional issues to be considered when using the fracture table were ensuring that Enid was securely positioned because of the potential movement during surgery and that she was covered to preserve her dignity at all times. Enid was positioned to avoid any damage to her skin from shearing forces. As recommended by Egol and Strauss (2009), a pressure-reducing foam mattress was used to reduce the possibility of damage to Enid's skin and deep tissue. Enid's non-dominant arm was secured on an arm board to allow access to her IV site. The other, which had the BP cuff applied, was placed alongside her body and secured using padded arm restraints. Her left leg was put into the fracture attachment stirrup, padded, secured and moved away from her mid plane to allow both surgical access and the C-arm access to take both a lateral and AP view. Her right leg was secured in the other fracture attachment stirrup. Enid's dignity was considered at all times during this positioning and it was ensured that her perineal area was covered at all times.

Prior to the surgical procedure starting, her positioning was checked to ensure that she was not touching any metal and that all the padding was still in place. In addition, all areas that could safely be covered were, and an adapted warming blanket was used to keep her temperature at an optimum level. Following confirmation from the anaesthetist that Enid's condition was stable, her left leg was prepared with a non-spirit-based antiseptic prep, twice to reduce the risk of infection. Normal standards of care were used in relation to swab, needle and instrument checks. Enid was then draped using sterile surgical drapes designed to provide optimum surgical access but also maximum barrier protection between the surgical site and the surrounding environment. These drapes came in a pack designed for this purpose.

4   **From the perspective of the ODP, consider the stages undertaken to repair a fractured neck of femur through using a dynamic hip screw.**

A   There is some debate as to whether an open or a minimally invasive technique is the preferred technique for DHS (Ho et al., 2009). Advantages of the minimally invasive technique include a shorter stay in hospital, reduced operative time, reduced infection rates and a reduction in blood loss, but these advantages need to be balanced against surgical expertise.

In Enid's case an open technique was used as this was considered normal practice. A small incision was made to gain access to the proximal femur and the DHS targeting device was introduced. This ensures that the guide wire is inserted at the correct angle for optimum reduction of the fracture. The guide wire was then introduced under x-ray control to stabilise the fracture. The DHS reamer and measuring device were then used to allow the introduction of the axial screw and plate. The plate was then fixed in place using screws. The axial screw and plate create compression to maximise reduction of the fracture and encourage healing. Following confirmation that all swabs, needles and instruments were accounted for, the wound was closed in layers using dissolvable sutures and, because of minimal blood loss, a drain was not used. Dissolvable sutures were the surgeon's preference as these reduced the possibility of further trauma to Enid's skin. A second check was performed by the scrubbed staff and all documentation was completed prior to preparing Enid for transfer into the PACU.

Enid's surgery took just over an hour and during this period she was kept sedated using ketamine, her temperature was monitored and warmed intravenous fluids were continued, in addition to continued monitoring of her pulse, oxygen saturation levels and blood pressure. Enid's temperature was monitored throughout the perioperative phase as recommended by the NICE (2008) *Guidelines*. This ensured that it did not drop below 36 degrees centigrade as this is considered to be hypothermia by Hamlin *et al.* (2009) and, if this occurs, it can have many effects on the homeostatic balance of the body, and can cause problems such as increased recovery times, increased wound infections and difficulty in managing pain – all of which could have extended Enid's hospital stay.

5 **What are Enid's postoperative care needs? This will include aspects of her transfer from the operating theatre to the PACU.**

A Enid was carefully moved from the fracture table, ensuring that her limbs and head were fully supported at all times as she was transferred on to her bed, which had been brought in from the PACU. Her dignity was ensured and the use of the warming blanket was continued. During this time Enid was reassured verbally prior to any procedure being carried out as the sedation was starting to wear off.

The scrub practitioner and the anaesthetist accompanied Enid to the PACU, where a full and comprehensive handover was carried out with the ODP who would continue Enid's care, before she went back to the ward. A full assessment was then carried out by the ODP using the ABCDE model: Airway, Breathing, Circulation, Disability and Exposure. In addition, Enid's pain was assessed on a continual basis using observation, communication and the hospital pain assessment tool. The hospital pain assessment tool was based on the 'visual analogue pain scale', which is recommended as being the most useful way of reporting pain by adult patients (Hatfield, 2014). The ODP regularly asked Enid how she was feeling, being aware that none of the pain assessment tools is perfect, and patient self-reporting is considered to be the most reliable guide to determine the type and nature of pain being experienced (Hamlin et al., 2009). As Enid's sedation wore off she said that she was not in pain but was uncomfortable and would like a cup of tea. Enid was encouraged to sit up in bed but was told she would have to wait until she got back to the ward before she could eat and drink.

Enid remained in the PACU until she was seen again by the anaesthetist, who checked on her progress with the PACU staff, and agreed that her sedation had worn off and her condition was considered stable. Pain assessment was continued and Enid was prescribed IV paracetamol for her pain. She was discharged to the ward and reassured that the surgeon would see her later on in the day. Enid was mobilised after physiotherapy review the same day as her surgery, as there were no other medical or surgical contraindications.

6 **Thinking about her overall patient experience, consider Enid's rehabilitation following her surgery.**

A Because of the early surgical intervention, and the availability of physiotherapy and occupational therapy to ensure that Enid mobilised early, her long-term recovery was very good, giving her the best possible opportunity to regain full mobility.

A number of issues have been identified for the longer-term rehabilitation of patients who have sustained hip fractures; these include early mobilisation, nutritional status and occupational therapy (Egol and Strauss, 2009; White et al., 2011). Egol and Strauss (2009) suggest that discharge planning should be coordinated, and Enid's discharge was discussed with her, her residential home provider, therapist and GP, and social support network (friends). Because she was local to the treatment centre and supported within her home environment she was discharged after six days, having met the requirements set out by the orthopaedic consultant and physiotherapist: being able to meet the basic living requirements and get up stairs with the use of crutches. As part of NICE (2011) hip fracture guidance, Enid's physiotherapy was continued on a daily basis until she was considered by physiotherapy review as mobile, but she was advised to attend regular outpatient review appointments.

REFERENCES AND FURTHER READING

Allman, K.G. and Wilson, I.H. (2011) *Oxford Handbook of Anaesthesia* (2nd edn). Oxford: Oxford University Press.

AO Foundation (2014) AO surgery reference. Available online at: www.aofoundation.org/surgery (accessed May 2014).

Association of Anaesthetists Great Britain and Ireland (AAGBI) (2012) *Checking Anaesthetic Equipment*. London: AAGBI.

Aveyard, H. and Sharp, P. (2013) *A Beginner's Guide to Evidence-Based Practice in Health and Social Care* (2nd edn). Maidenhead. Open University Press.

Barrett, D., Wilson, B. and Woollands, A. (2012) *Care Planning: A Guide for Nurses* (2nd edn). Pearson: Harlow.

Egol, K. and Strauss, J. (2009) Perioperative considerations in geriatric patients with hip fracture: what is the evidence? *Journal of Orthopaedic Trauma*, **23**(6): 386–394.

Fellows, S. and Fellows, B. (2012) *Paramedics: From Street to Emergency Department. Case Book*. Maidenhead: Open University Press.

Hamlin, L., Richardson-Tench, M. and Davies, M. (2009) *Perioperative Nursing: An Introductory Text*. London: Mosby Elsevier.

Hatfield, A. (2014) *The Complete Recovery Book* (4th edn). Oxford: Oxford University Press.

Ho, M., Garau, G., Walley, G., Oliva, F., Panni, A.S., Longo, U.L. and Maffulli, N. (2009) Minimally invasive dynamic hip screw for fixation of hip fractures. *International Orthopaedics*, **33**: 555–560.

Melia, K. (2014) *Ethics for Nursing and Healthcare Practice*. London: Sage.

National Institute for Health and Clinical Excellence (NICE) (2008) *Inadvertent Perioperative Hypothermia: The Management of Inadvertent Perioperative Hypothermia in Adults*. London: NICE.

National Institute for Health and Clinical Excellence (NICE) (2011) Hip fracture the management of hip fracture in adults. *NICE Clinical Guideline 124*. London: NICE.

National Institute for Health and Clinical Excellence (NICE) (2012) Osteoporosis: assessing the risk of fragility fracture. *NICE Clinical Guideline*. London: NICE.

NHS Institute for Innovation and Improvement (2013) *The Productive Operating Theatre*. London: Matrix Decisions Ltd.

White, J., Khan. W. and Smitham, P. (2011) Perioperative implications of surgery in elderly patients with hip fractures: an evidence based review. *Journal of Perioperative Practice*, **21**(6): 192–197.

Evacuation of retained products of conception: the care of Elizabeth Hugh
Adele Millington

INTRODUCTION AND LEARNING OUTCOMES

This case study details the perioperative care given to Elizabeth, a 35-year-old female undergoing evacuation of retained products of conception following a miscarriage at ten weeks' gestation. In addition to the surgical intervention, it is important that the psychological care of the patient be considered, and this case study will explore all aspects of Elizabeth's care.

By the end of this case study you will be able to:

- compare and contrast the different approaches to anaesthesia used to enable the patient to safely undergo an evacuation of retained products of conception (ERPC)
- discuss the advantages and disadvantages associated with different anaesthetic techniques
- undertake an appraisal of the physical and psychological care of the patient undergoing ERPC.

Case outline

Elizabeth Hugh is a 35-year-old who presented to theatre for evacuation of retained products of conception (ERPC) following a dating scan at ten weeks' gestation, which showed that a miscarriage had taken place; this is defined as the presence of a non-viable embryo/foetus (Wagaarachchi et al., 2001). In this case the miscarriage was asymptomatic, with the scan being the first indication of the problem.

Prior to this scan Elizabeth had seen her general practitioner (GP) for confirmation of the pregnancy and referral for booking with a midwife. During booking at eight weeks' gestation, past medical/surgical and obstetric history was established. Elizabeth had previously had minor surgical procedures, which had had no impact on previous pregnancies. However, her previous obstetric history included early stages of pre-eclampsia, and foetal bradycardia, which led to induction of labour and artificial rupture of membranes. Also an inappropriate foetal lie, for which intrauterine manipulation was unsuccessfully attempted and which resulted in severe foetal bradycardia, leading to a category-one Caesarean section.

1   Given Elizabeth's complicated maternal history, what other factors might it be important to establish prior to any surgery?

A   It was established that Elizabeth has a type 4 latex allergy, which is caused by a delayed immunological reaction. While not a life-threatening condition, this can cause severe itching and discomfort for the individual (Allergy UK, 2012). Although a potential problem, Elizabeth commented that her reaction was not severe.

Baseline observations were also established, including a BMI of 32. A healthy range for BMI is considered to be a maximum of 24.9, with a BMI of 32 falling into the obese range (Vorvick, 2014), which could impact on both Elizabeth's and her baby's health. In pregnancy a high BMI can result in the development of diabetes, high blood pressure, urinary tract infections, pelvic joint pain and DVT. Baseline blood pressure was also established, urine tested for protein, and blood taken for haemoglobin and to establish blood group. Due to Elizabeth's age, the midwife made the decision to refer for a slightly earlier dating scan to allow for any additional screening to be discussed and evaluated should this be required. The Royal College of Obstetricians and Gynaecologists (RCOG) (2009) states that, with a maternal age of over 35, there is an increased risk of miscarriage and adverse pregnancy outcomes; these increase with age, with those over 40 being at higher risk.

The date for this scan was arranged for approximately ten weeks' gestation. Unfortunately, following the scan, it was established that the viability of the pregnancy had ended at approximately eight weeks. Elizabeth and Mark (her husband) were given some time alone prior to a discussion about various options and then going home to consider the next steps. Elizabeth made the decision to undergo a surgical procedure in preference to medical management, which uses drugs to aid the expulsion of retained products, or expectant management, which allows the spontaneous passage of retained products of conception (Trinder *et al*., 2006). A date was arranged to attend for preoperative assessment and later for surgery.

2   What assessments are required preoperatively?

A   Preoperative assessment confirmed that baseline observations remained within normal range, and blood results for haemoglobin (Hb) and group were obtained. Hb in women is known to be lower in all ranges (Radford, Evans, and Williamson, 2011) and in pregnancy there is the potential for dilutional anaemia due to physiological changes, however this is usually at a later stage of pregnancy. As surgery increases the demand for oxygen, it is essential that oxygen-carrying capacity be maximised. It is necessary to know the woman's blood group as prophylactic anti-D should be given following miscarriage in women who are rhesus negative (Parker *et al*., 2006).

Stop and think

What information would Elizabeth need in order to help her prepare for her operation?

The procedure was discussed, supporting literature supplied and fasting times explained. Elizabeth was allowed to eat until 02.00 hours and able to drink clear fluids until 06.00 hours on the day of surgery. This is an attempt to reduce regurgitation and the possible risk of aspiration, which is multiplied with an increased BMI, which in turn can increase the risk of intra-abdominal pressure. It should be noted that the risk of aspiration increases in later pregnancy due to physiological changes; this is explored further in Case Study 8 (C-section).

As well as details of the procedure, information on various support groups and on future pregnancies was also made available to Elizabeth. Consent was not obtained at the preoperative visit as the health professional providing treatment was not present to discuss the benefits and risks of surgery (DH, 2009). However, consent was obtained on the day of surgery during the surgeon's preoperative visit, where the procedure, and its benefits and risks, were explained.

---

3 **Why is it important to discuss the disposal of the products of conception?**

A The issue of disposal of the products of conception was also discussed, and Elizabeth and her partner Mark were made aware of the local disposal policy and that there were options available should they wish for the tissue to be disposed of in a specific way. They were informed that they could delay this decision for a little while until they were ready. The Royal College of Nursing (RCN) (2007) suggests that 'parents should be given the same choice on the disposal of foetal remains as for a stillborn child'. They also recognise that at the time of loss parents may not wish to be involved but may request information about disposal at a later date, highlighting the need for good record keeping. Elizabeth and Mark made the decision to have the tissue disposed of by the hospital in whatever way was used and did not require further information about disposal.

4 **How was the operating theatre prepared in readiness for Elizabeth's operation?**

A Due to Elizabeth's latex allergy she was scheduled first on the theatre list; while many theatres today aim to provide a latex-free environment, there are still some items, such as sterile gloves, that in order to provide optimum tactility and protection are still more effective if made from latex (Aldyami *et al.*, 2010). However, in readiness for Elizabeth's operation, all latex products should ideally be removed from theatre, or if this is not possible, covered to prevent contact or aerolisation of latex (Kilgour and Mozdzen, 2014).

For this procedure to take place Elizabeth needs to be positioned in the lithotomy position, using lithotomy poles with gel-padded foot stirrups to prevent unnecessary pressure on the soles of the feet or behind the heels. Alternatively, Lloyd Davies poles could be used if the patient has problems with hip adduction or knee flexion (Knight and Mahajan, 2004).

Preparation for surgery includes the availability of a dilatation and curettage instrument set, which includes a uterine sound, Hegar dilators of various increasing sizes, curettes, polyp forceps, sponge holders, and both Vulsellum and Sims specula. In addition, there should be available wide-bore suction tubing, as well as a selection of flexible and rigid curettes of various sizes. The size of curette is determined following bimanual examination; this in turn determines the degree of cervical dilation, uterine fundal position and uterine size (Yancey, 2014). The choice of curette is determined by uterine axis and/or the surgeon's preference (Yancey, 2014).

5   **What different anaesthetic interventions could be used in order to undertake an ERPC?**

A   There are several forms of anaesthesia/analgesia that can be used to enable ERPC to be carried out, which include light sedation and paracervical block. Light sedation involves the intravenous injection of an anxiolytic and narcotic that, while enabling the patient to remain conscious and communicate, can also present some complications including respiratory depression. That said, the airway can still be compromised where a higher dose of sedation is used (Castleman and Mann, 2009).

Paracervical block involves the injection of local anaesthetic to anaesthetise nearby nerves (Tangsiriwatthana, Sankomkamhang and Lumbiganon, 2013). However, in a review of various methods of analgesia compared to paracervical block in uterine surgery, the evidence was inconclusive as to whether this kind of block is more effective for pain relief than other forms of local anaesthesia or sedation. Tangsiriwatthana *et al.* (2013: 2) suggest that 'women are likely to consider the rates and severity of pain during uterine interventions when performed awake to be unacceptable in the absence of neuraxial blockade'.

A further alternative is the use of a regional block in the form of spinal anaesthesia. This produces a rapid and dense anaesthesia, but an anaesthetic level of at least T8 is recommended (the level of T10 in some circumstances is thought to be insufficient to prevent pain during fundus manipulation or curettage) (Yentis and Malhotra, 2013). In experienced hands, spinal anaesthesia can be almost as fast acting as general anaesthesia. There are however instances where spinal anaesthesia is contraindicated, such as in patients with hypovolemia, systemic sepsis and coagulation disorders (Yentis and Malhotra, 2013). When preparing to use regional anaesthesia, consideration must be also given to the patient's emotional state, as the sights, sounds and smell of the operating theatre could be a distressing environment, especially for women who have recently experienced the bereavement of losing their baby.

In Elizabeth's case what can be considered a 'standard' general anaesthetic for ERPC was administered, consisting of propofol 2 mg/kg as the induction agent, with sevoflurane used to maintain anaesthesia, with both being viewed to support rapid recovery (BNF, 2009). It should be noted that high concentrations of inhalational agents should be avoided as this can lead to uterine relaxation, which can in turn lead to increased bleeding (Castleman and Mann, 2009). Fentanyl 50 mcg was given to support intraoperative pain relief. Because of the rapid nature of the surgery, postoperative pain diminishes quickly after the procedure, therefore opiate analgesia with a longer action is not required (Castleman and Mann, 2009).

A laryngeal mask airway (LMA) was used, despite Elizabeth's high BMI and the use of the lithotomy position, both of which factors can increase the risk of aspiration. Keller *et al.* (2004) suggest that assessment of aspiration risk is critical when determining whether LMA should be used. This assessment involves questioning the patient about upper gastrointestinal disease, which focuses on current symptoms and treatment (Keller *et al.*, 2004). It is suggested that most anaesthetists would consider that the LMA is contraindicated in patients with gastroesophageal reflux. However, a survey of anaesthetists revealed that up to 73% would use an LMA on such patients, or those with oesophagitis or hiatus hernia, provided it was asymptomatic (Crilly and McLeod, 2000).

On preoperative assessment Elizabeth presented with no history indicating oesophageal reflux or hiatus hernia. While there are potential risks associated with the use of LMA, which can potentially be exacerbated by a raised BMI, and the position required for surgery, overall these were balanced against the potential risks associated with endotracheal intubation (Divatia and Bhowmick, 2005), and indeed the overall shortness of the procedure.

6   **How would you describe the various stages carried out during a surgical ERPC?**

A   Elizabeth underwent a surgical evacuation of retained products of conception using a flexible aspiration cannula rather than the alternative rigid aspiration cannula. Kulier *et al.* (2001) found that, statistically, there was no difference between these in regard to incomplete or repeat uterine evacuation. The use of a flexible cannula throughout the first trimester has been advocated (Borgatta, Kattan and Stubblefield, 2012), however the same authors also note that in the United States there is a preference for the use of a rigid vacuum cannula as this allows the operator to view the products of conception as they are aspirated, indicating that the curette has been properly placed in the uterine cavity.

In order to insert the vacuum cannula most women require some cervical dilation. There are some exceptions in women who have a very early pregnancy (less than six weeks), or who already have a dilated cervix following spontaneous miscarriage (Borgatta *et al.*, 2012). Cervical dilation can also be achieved pharmaceutically using a prostaglandin analogue, which is the same as used in the medical management of evacuation of retained products of conception. If this is administered approximately three hours prior to surgery, mechanical dilation can be completely avoided and, if it is needed, it is technically easier because the cervix is softened. Administration of a prostaglandin analogue results in uterine contractions, and softening and dilation of the cervix (Borgatta *et al.*, 2012).

For Elizabeth's procedure cervical dilation was achieved manually using Hegar dilators. Hulka (2008) states that dilation of the internal os should proceed slowly, allowing the fibres of the internal os to stretch over the dilator for several seconds. If this is done too rapidly it can lead to tearing of these fibres. There is also the risk of forceful perforation of the uterus when resistance is overcome, and the technique should be adapted to reduce the risk of this (Hulka, 2008).

7   **What actions are required as part of Elizabeth's care once the surgical intervention is completed?**

A   Once surgery is complete a sanitary towel is placed over the vaginal area, as there is a potential for vaginal bleeding or a brownish discharge for up to two weeks post-surgery. This can be heavier than a normal period, but varies between individuals.

 While Elizabeth was being transferred to the post-anaesthetic care unit (PACU) the surgical team ensured that the foetal tissue was appropriately labelled. The theatre team must be aware of the requirements for the disposal of human tissue to ensure they do not contravene the patient's wishes and remain within the law. If parents have not agreed to histological examination of the foetal tissue there is no requirement for a separate specimen and all tissue can remain together to be disposed of as per the parents' wishes.

 Elizabeth was monitored thoroughly throughout her postoperative recovery. Careful consideration was also given to any vaginal blood loss – while it is expected there will be some bleeding, the amount varies from patient to patient.

8   **What specific assessments were undertaken in the post-anaesthetic care unit (PACU)?**

A   Following ERPC, Elizabeth was monitored for any postoperative pain, which is often described as 'period type' pain or uterine cramps, which diminish quickly after the procedure (Castleman and Mann, 2009). When Elizabeth was asked to rate her pain using a numerical rating score (with 0 being no pain and 10 being the worst imaginable pain), she scored her pain at 0.

 Elizabeth was also asked about nausea and she replied that she did not experience any postoperative nausea. However, because she had two or more risks factors associated with PONV this meant an 80% likelihood of her experiencing some PONV. With this in mind, ondansatron 4 mg was given intraoperatively, which has been shown to be twice as effective as metoclopramide in the treatment of PONV following gynaecological surgery (Hatfield, and Tronson, 2009). Furthermore, Wang et al. (2005) found that fewer patients who received ondansatron needed rescue medication in comparison to those who received other anti-emetics, such as dolasetron or granisetron. The same authors also noted that the patient's length of stay in the recovery room was significantly reduced when associated with the use of ondansatron. It should be noted – although this wasn't the case for Elizabeth – that PONV can also be triggered by oxytocic drugs such as Syntocinon, which is used to facilitate uterine evacuation and prevent post-procedural bleeding.

9   **Following the immediate postoperative phase, what are the longer-term implications for Elizabeth's recovery?**

A   Following this procedure, physical recovery is dependent on the individual. Recovery can be very quick, with only light to moderate bleeding for up to two weeks, or it can take a little longer. During this time patients such as Elizabeth are advised to use only sanitary towels and not tampons as there is potential for postoperative infection. Bleeding following ERPC is normal, so long as it does not become heavier than a normal period or begin to smell offensive (again a sign of infection). During this time it is possible that there will be some period-type pain but, again, over-the-counter analgesics such as paracetamol or ibuprofen normally suffice.

As Elizabeth had a general anaesthetic she was advised not to drive as many insurance companies do not provide cover for 48 hours post-anaesthetic; however this should be checked with individual companies (Bowden, 2010). Physical exercise can be resumed as soon as the individual feels ready, but activity such as swimming is best limited until after bleeding has stopped. Sexual intercourse can be resumed as soon as the couple feel ready, but it is advisable to abstain until bleeding has stopped to avoid further risk of infection.

Trying for another baby is at the discretion of the couple involved and there is no specific guidance, although it is often advised to wait until after a normal period – this, however, is ultimately the couple's decision. Bowden (2010) notes that there is no evidence to suggest that the length of time waited before sexual intercourse is resumed will have any significant impact on future pregnancies. While physically there are no limits, there may be emotional limitations for one or both partners, but this requires discussion between the couple themselves.

10 Consider Elizabeth's psychological recovery following her experience, and the care she and her husband may require.

A Psychological recovery following pregnancy loss may take longer than physical recovery, and while in Elizabeth's case there was a strong supportive network at home and external support was not required it was made clear that this was available should it be needed. Elizabeth was given information about counselling services and how to access these should they be required. Elizabeth was also given information about the remembrance book should she wish to make an entry of remembrance, and was supplied with information about the remembrance garden should she wish to visit it.

In Elizabeth's case there was very little obvious consideration of Mark's emotional state, although he was involved with Elizabeth's care throughout, which was the choice of the couple. Having a private room throughout Elizabeth's hospital stay enabled her husband to be with her throughout, and to be involved in conversations with the consultant and nursing staff about anticipated events and potential future pregnancies. However, if Elizabeth had not wanted her husband involved then staff would have had to adhere to her wishes. In this instance Elizabeth is the patient that needs consideration and it is her decision as to what information is shared with a third party; staff are bound by confidentiality and, unless explicitly stated, issues around care can be discussed only with the patient. This may raise some issues with the partner, but these have to be resolved between the couple and explained.

Telling friends and family was the most difficult aspect of this experience for Elizabeth and her husband. Although still in the very early stages of pregnancy it had been necessary to tell some family members about it to enable help with childcare during pregnancy-related hospital appointments and scans to be arranged. Also it was necessary to tell some friends and work colleagues, to explain physical changes that required some adaptation. While everyone who knew Elizabeth and her husband were very supportive and understanding it was difficult for some time, even after returning to work. Fortunately Elizabeth and Mark had made the decision not to tell their first child until a lot later in the pregnancy and this meant they did not have to explain what had happened to a young child.

Healthcare professionals were generally supportive and prepared to listen to the thoughts and opinions of Elizabeth, and appeared quite sensitive to the family's needs, particularly those involved in the hospital care of the family. However, there were some who used platitudes to explain away the pregnancy loss such as 'something went wrong early in the pregnancy', which may have been the case, but is only one possible cause of pregnancy loss and does not offer a definitive answer for Elizabeth and her family. As Yentis and Malhotra (2013) state, this procedure may be considered a minor one by healthcare staff, but for the mother it may be the loss of a much wanted baby. For Elizabeth and Mark, this was a much wanted pregnancy, and staff involved in Elizabeth's care were very supportive. In the operating theatre, in addition to the grieving process, Elizabeth was in an alien environment, which was also quite frightening, and staff were required to be very supportive prior to anaesthesia and after the procedure.

REFERENCES AND FURTHER READING

Aldyami, E., Kulkarni, A., Reed, M.R. and Scott, D.M. (2010) Latex free gloves: safer for whom? *Journal of Arthroplasty*, **25**(1): 27–30.

Allergy UK (2012) Rubber latex allergy. Available online at: www.allergyuk.org/rubber-latex-allergy/rubber-latex-allergy (accessed 7 October 2015).

Apfel, C.C., Laara, E., Koivuranta, M. *et al.* (1999) A simplified risk score for predicting post operative nausea and vomiting: conclusions from cross-validations between two centres, in Hatfield, A. and Tronson, M. (eds) *The Complete Recovery Room Book* (4th edn). Oxford: Oxford University Press.

Borgatta, L., Kattan, D. and Stubblefield, P.G. (2012) *Surgical Techniques for First Trimester Abortion*. London: Foundation for the Global Library of Women's Medicine.

Bowden, P. (2010) Advice following a miscarriage. Basingstoke and North Hampshire NHS Foundation Trust. Available online at: hampshirehospitals.nhs.uk (accessed 16 July 2014).

British National Formulary (BNF) (2009) *BNF 57*. London: BMJ Group.

Castleman, L. and Mann, C. (2009) *Manual Vacuum Aspiration (MVA) for Uterine Evacuation: Pain Management* (2nd edn). Chapel Hill, NC: Ipas.

Crilly, H. and McLeod, K. (2000) Use of the laryngeal mask airway – a survey of Australian anaesthetic practice. *Anaesthetic Intensive Care*, **28**: 224.

Department of Health (DH) (2009) *Reference Guide to Consent for Examination or Treatment* (2nd edn). Available online at: www.gov.uk/government/uploads/system/uploads/attachment_data/file/138296/dh_103653__1_.pdf (accessed 14 July 2014).

Divatia, J.V. and Bhowmick, K. (2005) Complications of endotracheal intubation and other airway management procedures. *Indian Journal of Anaesthesia*, **49**: 308–318.

Hatfield, A. and Tronson, M. (2009) *The Complete Recovery Room Book* (4th edn). Oxford: Oxford University Press.

Hulka, J. (2008) *Dilatation and Curettage*. London: Foundation for the Global Library of Women's Medicine.

Keller, C., Brimacombe, J., Bittersohl, J., Lirk, P. and Von Goedecke, A. (2004) Aspiration and the laryngeal mask airway: three cases and a review of the literature. *British Journal of Anaesthesia*, **93**(4): 579–582.

Kilgour, J. and Mozdzen, K. (2014) Working towards latex safe environments (contact and airborne transmission) prevention and management. Available online at: www.wrha.mb.ca/professionals/familyphysicians/files/WorkingLatexSafeEnvirons.pdf (accessed 7 October 2015).

Knight, D.J.W. and Mahajan, R.P. (2004) Patient positioning in anaesthesia. *Continuing Education in Anaesthesia, Critical Care and Pain*, **4**(5): 160–163.

Kulier, R., Cheng, L., Fekih, A., Hofmeyr, G.J. and Campana, A. (2001) Surgical methods for first trimester termination of pregnancy. *Cochrane Database of Systematic Reviews*. Issue 4.

National Institute for Health and Clinical Excellence (NICE) (2008) *Inadvertent Perioperative Hypothermia: The Management of Inadvertent Perioperative Hypothermia in Adults*. London: NICE.

Parker, J., Wray, J., Gooch, A., Robson, S. and Qureshi, H. (2006) Guidelines for the use of prophylactic anti-D immunoglobulin. British Committee for Standards in Haematology. Available online at: www.bcshguidelines.com/documents/Anti-D_bcsh_07062006.pdf (accessed 10 July 2014).

Radford, M., Evans, C. and Williamson, A. (2011) *Perioperative Assessment and Perioperative Management*. Keswick: M&K Publishing.

Royal College of Nursing (RCN) (2007) *Sensitive Disposal of all Foetal Remains: Guidance for Nurses and Midwives*. London: Royal College of Nursing.

Royal College of Obstetricians and Gynaecologists (RCOG) (2009) RCOG statement on later maternal age. Available online at: www.rcog.org.uk/en/news/rcog-statement-on-later-maternal-age (accessed 16 July 2014).

Tangsiriwatthana, T., Sankomkamhang, U.S. and Lumbiganon, M. (2013) Paracervical local anaesthesia for cervical dilatation and uterine intervention. *Cochrane Database of Systematic Reviews 2013*. Issue 9: 2.

Trinder, J., Brocklehurst, P., Porter, R., Read, M., Vyas, S. and Smith, L. (2006) Management of miscarriage: expectant, medical or surgical? Results of randomised controlled trial (miscarriage treatment (MIST) trial). *British Medical Journal*, **332**(7552): 1235–1240.

Vorvick, L.J. (2014) Body mass index. Available online at: www.nlm.nih.gov/medlineplus/ency/article/007196.htm (accessed 7 October 2015).

Wagaarachchi, P.T., Ashok, P.W., Narvekar, N., Smith, N.C. and Templeton, A. (2001) Medical management of early fetal demise using a combination of mifepristone and misoprostol. *Human Reproduction*, **16**(9): 1849–1853.

Wang, S., Grece, J., Joseph, R.A., Feuerman, M. and Malone, B. (2005) Evaluation of three 5-HT3 receptor antagonists in the prevention of postoperative nausea and vomiting in adults. *Pharmacy and Therapeutics*, **30**: 341–353.

Yancey, J.D. (2014) Dilation and curettage with suction. Available online at: http://emedicine.medscape.com/atricle/1848296-overview#a15 (accessed 7 July 2014).

Yentis, S. and Malhotra, S. (2013) *Analgesia, Anaesthesia and Pregnancy* (3rd edn). Cambridge: Cambridge University Press.

Inguinal hernia repair: the care of Matthew Senior

Fiona Ritchie

INTRODUCTION AND LEARNING OUTCOMES

This case study examines the care given to a 48-year-old male patient undergoing repair of left inguinal hernia. The case study considers the holistic care of the patient from the outpatient clinic to discharge home, and includes specific considerations of the patient's perioperative journey.

By the end of this case study you will be able to:

- explain the implications of hernia repair surgery for the patient and their family
- discuss the holistic care requirements of a patient undergoing hernia repair and, in particular, their perioperative care needs
- describe evidence-based, safe and effective care, from hospital to home, for patients undergoing inguinal hernia repair.

Case outline

Matthew Senior is a 48-year-old male who lives with his wife and three children, aged 18, 16 and 10, in a three-bedroom, ground-floor flat. He is a self-employed bricklayer and at the time of surgical referral was working on a project with a guarantee of a further nine months' work. He is an ex-smoker who smoked 20 cigarettes a day until five years ago. Mr Senior was referred to the general surgical clinic following an appointment with his GP. At the general surgical outpatient clinic he described having 'a lump in his left groin', which was increasing in size and was beginning to cause him pain in the left groin and scrotal region. He described being able to 'pop the lump back in', however this was becoming increasingly difficult to achieve. He stated that the lump would 'pop out' at work, often when lifting or straining.

---

1 **How might you define an abdominal hernia?**

A Matthew was examined by the consultant surgeon, who made the diagnosis of left inguinal hernia. A broad definition of abdominal hernia is 'the projection of a peritoneal lined sac through a weakness in the abdominal wall' (Rothrock, 2011). Abdominal herniae occur most frequently in males, with the majority being indirect inguinal hernia. An indirect inguinal hernia is where abdomen contents have protruded through the inguinal ring, in contrast to a direct hernia where the abdominal contents have protruded through an area of weakness in the transversus abdominus and transversalis fascia (Rothrock, 2011).

2 **Other than surgery, how else might Matthew be treated?**

A It was explained to Matthew that the options were either conservative or surgical treatment. Conservative treatment would mean living with the hernia and making lifestyle changes, including the avoidance of heavy lifting, which could prove difficult due to the nature of his occupation. It was also explained that, with conservative treatment, his symptoms would not be completely resolved, the hernia may increase in size, the hernia may become irreducible, and that there was a possibility that the hernia may become strangulated and require emergency surgery to prevent or alleviate a bowel obstruction. It was then explained that, if surgery were the chosen option, it would involve a traditional open approach as a unilateral inguinal hernia did not meet the criteria for minimal access surgery, as determined by his particular National Health Service (NHS) provider. In order to meet the criteria for minimal access inguinal hernia repair surgery, the hernia must be either recurrent or bilateral.

Stop and think

What other information should Matthew be provided with in order to make an informed choice about his treatment?

The patient was informed that a synthetic mesh would be implanted and used to reinforce the defect, thereby preventing abdominal contents from protruding. The benefits and risks of surgery were explained to him including, in the short term, the possibility of wound infection, bruising, swelling, numbness, pain and discomfort, deep vein thrombosis, pulmonary embolism and urinary retention. In the long term there are risks of chronic pain, mesh infection and hernia recurrence (Rothrock, 2011). After considering his options, Matthew elected to undergo surgical treatment to repair his left inguinal hernia.

---

3 **Which pre-assessment activities were carried out prior to surgical intervention, paying particular attention to any pre-existing medical conditions?**

A Immediately following his consultation, Matthew was taken to the pre-assessment clinic, and assessed for his suitability for day case surgery and anaesthesia. He was assessed to ensure that he met the Association of Anaesthetists of Great Britain and Ireland (AAGBI) guidelines for day case and short stay surgery (AAGBI, 2011). The AAGBI guidelines recommend that social, medical and surgical factors be taken into account when assessing suitability for ambulatory care.

A full medical history was taken by the clinic nurse and it was noted that Mr Senior has a BMI of 29, and suffers from stable angina and gastroesophageal reflux disease (GORD). In accordance with the Scottish Intercollegiate Guidelines Network (2007), he is currently prescribed a beta blocker for stable angina. He is taking the drug atenalol 100 mg once per day and has a glyceryl trinitrate (GTN) spray, from which he sprays one dose, once or twice, under his tongue for symptom relief. Beta blockers are used for patients with stable angina as they cause a decrease in heart rate and cardiac contractility, thereby reducing stress on the heart, which can prevent or reduce the frequency of angina episodes. Matthew is prescribed a proton pump inhibitor (PPI) and omeperazole 20 mg once per day to alleviate the symptoms of GORD. Proton pump inhibitors reduce the secretion of gastric acid in the stomach and decrease the symptoms of GORD by lessening the amount of acid flowing into the oesophagus. Matthew's angina occurs infrequently, and only during periods of strenuous exertion or exercise. During pre-assessment, blood samples were taken for analysis of urea and electrolytes, and for a full blood count. Matthew had a 12-lead electrocardiograph (ECG) carried out, which demonstrated no recent changes and therefore a request for follow-up exercise tolerance test, echocardiogram or referral to a cardiologist were not required.

4   **What specific criteria were used to ascertain whether Matthew was suitable for day surgery?**

A   The following should be present.

- Matthew fully understood what was going to happen throughout the planned procedure.
- He had an escort home, who would provide him with assistance in the 24 hours following surgery.
- In spite of the presence of angina it was stable and being successfully managed by medication.
- The planned surgery did not carry significant risk of complications necessitating urgent medical intervention.
- Analgesia could be achieved by oral medication.
- Oral intake could be resumed within a few hours of surgery.

Following this, arrangements were made for Matthew's future admission to the ambulatory care hospital.

5   **How would the perioperative team have specifically prepared for Matthew's care in the operating theatre?**

A   On the day of surgery, the risks, benefits and alternative treatment options for inguinal hernia were again explained to the patient. Matthew stated that he wished to proceed with the surgery and gave his written consent. He was visited by the consultant anaesthetist, who explained that the results of the blood samples taken at the clinic were within normal limits. The option of a spinal anaesthetic was discussed, however this was declined and a general anaesthetic was requested. Matthew explained that he felt very uncomfortable about a spinal anaesthetic as he was anxious about undergoing surgery and wanted to be 'asleep'. It was explained to him that sedation could be administered, which would reduce his awareness during surgery, however he declined this option. The patient reported that his GORD was not currently well controlled in spite of regularly using the proton pump inhibitor, and it was therefore decided that endotracheal intubation would be carried out using a rapid sequence induction (RSI) technique. This would be undertaken to minimise the risk of aspiration of stomach contents (Aitkenhead, Moppett and Thompson, 2013). The procedure was explained to the patient, who also reported that following a previous general anaesthetic to repair a hand laceration he had suffered from postoperative nausea and vomiting (PONV). The anaesthetist explained that he would administer medication that should help prevent this happening. An airway assessment was carried out, which gave no indication that a difficult airway was anticipated.

On the day of surgery a team brief (NHS Scotland, 2012) was carried out prior to the start of the operating list, and each patient and their individual care needs discussed. Following team introductions, the team discussed Matthew's care, during which the anaesthetist informed the perioperative team that he would be carrying out a rapid sequence induction, however there were no other anticipated airway issues and that he intended to carry out an ilio-inguinal nerve block for postoperative analgesia. He also informed the perioperative team that Matthew was allergic to penicillin.

The surgeon gave an account of the patient's medical history and that she intended to carry out a Lichtenstein, tension-free mesh repair, and gave a list of the sutures she intended to use, and the anticipated type and size of mesh required. It was confirmed that the sutures and mesh required were available, and a variety of alternative sizes and types of mesh were also available. The surgeon requested a basic tray of general surgical instruments and a self-retaining retractor with long prongs. The surgeon stated that she did not anticipate that antibiotics would be required, as recommended by the British Hernia Society (2013), and that the anticipated blood loss was minimal. Matthew had anti-embolism stockings in situ and would not require the use of an electrical intermittent pneumatic compression device for prevention of deep venous thrombosis. At this point the team stated that they did not require any further information in order to proceed to the anaesthetic stage.

6 **How would you ensure the safe care of Matthew during induction of anaesthesia?**

A Prior to the rapid sequence induction (RSI) the anaesthetist and those providing skilled assistance planned for the intervention (preparation included drugs, equipment, people and place). Consideration was also given to the position and protection of the cervical spine given the hyperextension needed to undertake RSI. The patient's trolley was checked to ensure the head down tilt was fully functioning, and suction was switched on and placed under the patient's pillow. A tape to tie the ET tube in place was placed under the patient's neck and a final set of observations were made, which were again within normal limits.

The anaesthetist described the action to be taken in the event of a difficult airway scenario, which followed the Difficult Airway Society Guidelines (Difficult Airway Society, 2004). An additional member of the theatre team, who was competent to perform cricoid pressure, was asked to undertake application of cricoid pressure in order to allow the anaesthetic practitioner to concentrate on providing skilled assistance to the anaesthetist.

Non-invasive monitoring was applied and a set of baseline observations carried out; these were noted to be within normal limits – heart rate was 82, blood pressure 137/82 and arterial oxygen saturation 97%. The ECG trace showed no abnormalities. A size 18 gauge cannula was inserted and an infusion of 500 ml of Hartmann's solution was commenced, to be infused over a period of two hours. Fentanyl, an opiate analgesic drug, was administered intravenously to provide analgesia and also assist with intubation as it dulls laryngeal reflexes. Matthew was pre-oxygenated to provide a reservoir of oxygen for the period of apnoea triggered by the administration of succinylcholine.

Pressure was applied to the cricoid cartilage at the rate of 10 N (Newtons) and the induction agent, in this case propofol, was given; when consciousness was lost, 30 N of pressure was applied (Aitkenhead *et al.*, 2013) and the neuromuscular blocking agent, suxamethonium, given. Suxamethonium is used due to its properties of rapid onset and short duration. When muscle fasciculations had ceased, laryngoscopy was performed and a good view of the vocal cords was achieved. A size 9.0 ET tube was inserted, and the cuff immediately inflated by the anaesthetic assistant. The patient was gently hand ventilated, and bilateral, even chest movement was noted as was moisture in the catheter mount and endotracheal tube. The capnography trace indicated that CO_2 was being exhaled by the patient. Following chest auscultation confirming air entry, the anaesthetist instructed that cricoid pressure could be removed. The patient continued to be hand ventilated until breathing resumed. As the patient had previously reported having experienced postoperative nausea and vomiting, he was given 4 mg of the anti-emetic drug ondansetron as a prophylactic measure at induction of anaesthesia.

7   **Matthew had consented to an ilio-inguinal nerve block as part of his anaesthetic. How was this undertaken?**

A   Matthew had consented to an ilio-inguinal nerve block for pain relief and this was carried out following the return of spontaneous breathing. An ilio-inguinal block is commonly used to provide analgesia following an inguinal hernia repair (McLeod, McCartney and Wildsmith, 2013). The anaesthetist initiated the 'STOP' moment to ensure the block was being correctly sited (Safe Anaesthesia Liaison Group, 2011). Immediately prior to inserting the block, the surgical site marking and the correct side were checked and confirmed with the anaesthetic assistant. A 35 mm, 21 gauge needle was used to penetrate the skin 1 cm medially and inferiorly to the anterior superior iliac spine. The needle was advanced at an angle of 90° until the external oblique was penetrated, and 8 ml of levobupivacaine 0.5% was injected to block the ilio-hypogastric nerve. The needle was further advanced and the internal oblique penetrated with a further 8 ml of levobupivacaine 0.5% injected to block the ilio-inguinal nerve.

8   **How would the perioperative team have specifically prepared for Matthew's care in the operating theatre?**

A   Matthew was attached to the breathing circuit and monitoring equipment, and anaesthesia was maintained using oxygen, nitrous oxide and a volatile agent. The patient was positioned on the operating table in the supine position, where arm boards were used to support his upper limbs and gel pads placed underneath his heels to mini-mise the risk of formation of pressure ulcers. Matthew was wearing compression stockings in order to minimise the risk of venous thromboembolism. A surgical pause (WHO, 2008) was carried out, which confirmed the following: patient's name, date of birth, unique patient identification number, procedure to be undertaken, confirmation of correct site marking, confirmation of written consent, absence of metal implants, that he was allergic to penicillin and that prophylactic antibiotics were not required.

The patient's temperature was monitored throughout the procedure, to promote normothermia, and an upper forced air warmer was used. The warmer settings were adjusted according to the temperature readings. The electrosurgery return electrode was applied to the patient's left thigh. Hair clipping was not required at the site of the return electrode, although clippers were used to remove excess hair from the left side of the abdomen immediately prior to preoperative skin preparation. Preoperative skin preparation was carried out using chlorhexadine gluconate 2% in 70% isopropyl alco-hol, and the area was allowed time to dry. Care was taken to avoid fluid spill on to the electrosurgical dispersive electrode as incomplete adherence to the chosen site may cause electrosurgery equipment to malfunction (Potty, Khan and Tailor, 2010). The area of skin preparation extended from the umbilicus to mid-thigh, and the surgical drapes were placed to minimise exposure while allowing for identification of anatom-ical landmarks and the possibility of the need to extend the incision. Sterile light handles were attached, and return and active electrode cables connected to the electrosurgical generator.

q   **Describe the basic surgical technique used to carry out an inguinal hernia repair?**

A   It is essential that the anaesthetist is made aware that an initial painful stimulus is about to be administered to the patient (knife to skin). This ensures that surgery does not commence until an adequate level of anaesthesia has been achieved. The incision was made at the pubic tubercle and extended to the mid-inguinal point. Sub-cutaneous fat, scarpa fascia and external oblique aponeurosis were opened, taking care to protect the ilio-inguinal nerve from injury. A self-retaining retractor with long, blunt prongs was used to expose the surgical site and was repositioned as layers were exposed, with haemostasis being maintained throughout. The spermatic cord and cremaster muscle were carefully contained in a Littlewood forcep and the presence of a hernia sac identified. Two artery forceps were used to assist with opening of cremaster muscle, and the sac separated from the cord and accom-panying structures.

The sac was opened, the abdominal contents were restored to the peritoneal cavity and a 2/0 gauge, braided absorbable purse-string suture was used to close the sac. A 15 x 8 cm polypropylene mesh was shaped to fit and used to repair the defect. Care was taken that excess fragments of mesh were not introduced into the wound. The polypropylene mesh was sutured into position using a 2/0 gauge monofilament, non-absorbable suture.

During closure of the layers the self-retaining retractor was repositioned to assist with visualisation of the surgical site. The external oblique aponeurosis and the scarpa fascia were repaired using a 1 gauge braided absorbable suture, an 'account-able items count' carried out and the result communicated to the surgeon. The skin was then repaired using a 3/0 gauge monofilament suture, with a final accountable items count carried out (AfPP, 2011) and again communicated to the surgeon.

As stipulated by the Health and Care Professions Council (2016) and Nursing and Midwifery Council (2015), the care delivered to the patient during anaesthesia and surgery was documented by the anaesthetic and circulating practitioners throughout and the care plan was checked at the end of the procedure, by the scrub practitioner, to ensure accuracy.

10   **Describe Matthew's handover and his immediate post-anaesthetic care.**

A   At the end of the procedure, while still in the operating theatre, the patient met the criteria for extubation. He was breathing spontaneously, blood pressure, pulse, respiratory rate, oxygen saturation and end tidal carbon dioxide ($ETCO_2$) were within normal limits, and protective reflexes had returned. With suction readily available, the endotracheal tube cuff was deflated and the endotracheal tube removed. Oxygen was then administered via an appropriate oxygen mask.

As Matthew's vital signs were within normal limits he was transferred to the post-anaesthetic care unit (PACU).

Stop and think

What information is needed to ensure a successful handover from the theatre team to the PACU?

The handover should include the following information:

- the patient's name and age
- surgical procedure
- anaesthetic type and the fact that a rapid sequence induction had been carried out
- an ilio-inguinal block had been inserted
- instructions for oxygen therapy
- past medical history, including previous incidence of postoperative nausea and vomiting
- drugs administered during surgery
- drugs prescribed for use in the PACU
- instructions on intravenous fluid replacement
- instruction that the patient may be allowed home if he meets the discharge criteria
- advice for the patient concerning analgesia on return home.

Immediately following the handover by the anaesthetist, the operating room practitioner communicated the following:

- confirmation of patient's name and procedure
- skin sutures used
- type of wound dressing
- temperature status during surgery
- pressure area and return electrode site skin status
- confirmation all necessary paperwork/case notes accompany patient.

---

11 **How would you prioritise Matthew's post-anaesthetic care?**

A The recovery practitioner undertook the Airway, Breathing, Circulation, Drugs/Drips/Dressings/Drains and Extras approach to caring for Matthew (Hatfield, 2014). Routine observations of blood pressure, pulse, oxygen saturation level, ECG tracing, respiratory rate, temperature, pain score and sedation score were carried out at 15-minute intervals, and more frequently if any deterioration was detected.

Throughout Matthew's stay in the PACU it was important to determine that his airway was clear and the head of the trolley was raised to assist with breathing. Had it been necessary, suction was available to clear the mouth and pharynx of secretions, taking care to avoid inducing laryngospasm (Hatfield, 2014). The oxygen saturation readings were consistently between 97% and 99%, which indicated that the patient was not hypoxic. The remaining Hartmann's solution was administered over the next 45 minutes (500 ml in total). The wound dressing was checked at each set of observations to ensure that there was no sign of haemorrhage, and throughout the recovery episode only slight blood spotting was observed.

12 **How was Matthew's postoperative pain monitored, recorded and managed?**

A The recovery practitioner used a numeric scale (using numbers 0–10) to rate Matthew's pain. He had reported a pain rating of 0 on arrival in the PACU, however after 15 minutes this had increased to a rating of 5. Matthew was reassured that his pain would be addressed and that analgesia would be given. The drug prescription chart and anaesthetic chart were checked to identify which analgesic drugs had been prescribed and determine if they had been given previously – and, if so, that the appropriate interval had elapsed prior to further administration. As no paracetamol had been given to the patient, 1 g of paracetamol was administered intravenously and the patient was again reassured. The patient's pain rating was reassessed regularly and, after 15 minutes, it reduced from a score of 5 to a score of 3; a further 15 minutes later it had reduced to 2.

The recovery practitioner noted that the patient did not show any signs of postoperative nausea and vomiting and therefore no further anti-emetic medication was required. The movement from stage one to stage two recovery was uneventful. The PACU care was recorded throughout on the patient care plan and a verbal handover given to the staff in the discharge lounge. Matthew's recovery was uneventful and he had a light snack and drink prior to being collected by his wife. He was able to pass urine without difficulty two hours post-surgery.

13 **Describe the longer-term aspects of Matthew's recovery following inguinal hernia repair.**

A Both Matthew and his wife were given verbal and written instructions of what to do and what to expect in terms of recovery following inguinal hernia surgery. Matthew's wife confirmed that she would care for him for the first 24 hours following surgery. The wound dressing was to be removed the following day, and thereafter baths or showers to be taken as normal. The wound was to be dried gently, and perfumes and products containing talcum powder were to be avoided. Matthew and his wife were advised that bruising may develop around the groin, scrotum and penis, and there may be some swelling. They were informed that this does not indicate that there has been a recurrence of the hernia but is a normal part of the wound healing process.

Absorbable sutures were used for skin closure and therefore did not need to be removed. Occasionally, the end of the suture can be seen and they were instructed that this is quite normal. Paracetamol/ibuprofen would provide adequate analgesia following discharge, however if this did not relieve the pain further medical advice should be sought.

Matthew was advised that driving could be resumed whenever he was able to change gear and make an emergency stop safely and comfortably. It was stressed that he must contact his car insurance company to confirm that his policy would allow him to return to driving. Constipation can occur following surgery and a gentle over-the-counter laxative may be required to help Matthew resume normal bowel habits. Drinking plenty of fluid will also help. Both Matthew and his wife were surprised to hear that an early return to normal activities is recommended and has been shown to benefit recovery following hernia repair (Bay-Nielsen *et al.*, 2004). They were re-assured that most patients are able to return to normal activities within a fortnight of surgery (Kurzer, Kark and Hussain, 2007) and the average patient should be expected to return to work within seven days, albeit with a restriction of two to three weeks for heavy lifting (British Hernia Society, 2013). The couple were also advised that they should seek medical attention if any of the following occurred:

- bruising and/or swelling that was more severe than had previously been described to them
- abdominal pain not resolved by recommended analgesia
- loss of appetite
- nausea and/or vomiting
- high temperature
- calf pain
- breathlessness
- difficulty passing urine.

They were given a 24-hour direct telephone number and advised to phone the day surgery unit if they had any further questions once discharged home.

Matthew returned home and made an uneventful recovery. He was able to return to work two weeks after surgery, however he refrained from heavy lifting for a further two weeks. Matthew had been concerned that his recent surgery could have jeopardised his employment and was relieved that he was able to resume work in such a short space of time.

REFERENCES AND FURTHER READING

Aitkenhead, A., Moppett, I. and Thompson, J. (2013) *Smith and Aitkenhead's Textbook of Anaesthesia* (6th edn). Edinburgh: Churchill Livingstone.

Association for Perioperative Practice (AfPP) (2011) *Standards and Recommendations for Safe Perioperative Practice* (3rd edn). Harrogate: AfPP.

Association of Anaesthetists of Great Britain and Ireland (AAGBI) (2011) Guidelines: day case and short stay surgery. Available online at: www.aagbi.org/sites/default/files/Day%20Case%20for%20web.pdf (accessed 2 May 2014).

Bay-Nielsen, M., Thomsen, H., Andersen, F. *et al*. (2004) Convalescence after inguinal herniorrhaphy. *British Journal of Surgery*, **91**(3): 362–367.

British Hernia Society (2013) Groin hernia guidelines. Available online at: www.britishherniasociety.org/hernia-guidelines-2/ (accessed 15 March 2014).

Difficult Airway Society (2004) Unanticipated difficult tracheal intubation during rapid sequence induction of anaesthesia in the non-obstetric adult patient. Available online at: www.das.uk.com/files/rsi-Jul04-A4.pdf (accessed 15 March 2014).

Hatfield, A. (2014) *The Complete Recovery Room Book* (5th edn). Oxford: Oxford University Press.

Health and Care Professions Council (2016) *Standards of Conduct, Performance and Ethics*. London: Health and Care Professions Council.

Kurzer, M., Kark, A. and Hussain, T. (2007) Inguinal hernia repair. *Journal of Perioperative Practice*, **17**(7): 318–330.

McLeod, G., McCartney, C. and Wildsmith, J. (2013) *Principles and Practice of Regional Anaesthesia* (4th edn). Oxford: Oxford University Press.

NHS Scotland Quality Improvement Hub (2012) Communications: surgical brief and pause. Available online at: www.qihub.scot.nhs.uk/quality-dimensions/safe/patient-safety-in-scotland/communications-surgical-brief-and-pause.aspx (accessed 22 February 2014).

Nursing and Midwifery Council (2015) *The Code: Professional Standards of Practice and Behaviour for Nurses and Midwives*. London: Nursing and Midwifery Council.

Potty, A., Khan, W. and Tailor, H. (2010) Diathermy in perioperative practice. *Journal of Perioperative Practice*, **20**(11): 402–405.

Rothrock, J.C. (2011) *Alexander's Care of the Patient in Surgery* (14th edn). Missouri: Elsevier.

Safe Anaesthesia Liaison Group (2011) 'Stop before you block' campaign. Available online at: www.rcoa.ac.uk/standards-of-clinical-practice/wrong-site-block (accessed 27 February 2014).

Saxena, P. (2013) Lichtenstein hernioplasty. Available online at: www.reference.medscape.com/article/1892759-overview (accessed 16 March 2014).

Scottish Intercollegiate Guidelines Network (2007) Management of stable angina. Available online at: www.sign.ac.uk/pdf/sign96.pdf (accessed 1 March 2014).

World Health Organization (WHO) (2008) Safe surgery saves lives. Available online at: www.who.int/patientsafety/safesurgery/knowledge_base/SSSL_Brochure_finalJun08.pdf (accessed 14 March 2014).

Tonsillectomy: the care of Ellie Brown

David Hughes

INTRODUCTION AND LEARNING OUTCOMES

Children account for approximately one-third of all patients undergoing ear, nose and throat (ENT) surgery. Tonsillectomy is one of the most frequently performed surgical operations in children, with 18,000 tonsillectomies performed in children less than 16 years of age in England in 2012 (RCS, 2013). With the improvement of technologies in anaesthetics and the advancement of surgery, at least 90% of surgery in children can now be performed on a day-stay basis (AAGBI, 2010: 19). This case study discusses the care attributed to one such child, Ellie Brown.

By the end of this case study you will be able to:

• explain the processes in place to facilitate a day case procedure
• summarise the physiological role the tonsils play in fighting infection as part of the immune system
• explore the holistic care of Ellie and the support offered to her mother
• explain the rationale for selected equipment and relevant pharmacology specific to a paediatric tonsillectomy patient.

Case outline

Ellie Brown is a 10-year-old girl who lives at home with her single-parent mum, Gail, and her older brother. She is normally a fit and healthy child, who enjoys reading, dancing and attending her weekly swimming lessons. Her 'personal child health record' presents details that, by the age of 5, Ellie had received all of her required immunisations against diphtheria, tetanus, polio, meningitis, measles, mumps and rubella. Her past medical history is relatively uneventful, with two occurrences of childhood illness, namely measles and chicken pox, both while Ellie was 6 years of age. Intermittently, over the past 12 months, she has been complaining of a sore throat, and feeling feverish with a raised temperature, which her mum had been treating with Calpol SixPlus. During these episodes of feeling unwell, Ellie has found it very difficult to swallow solid foods while eating her meals. The latter was discussed between Ellie's mum and her class teacher during a parents' evening at Ellie's primary school, as her teacher had also noticed a change in Ellie's eating habits during school lunchtime periods and had enquired if everything was fine at home. These episodes of sickness have resulted in Ellie missing a number of days of school over the past 12 months. Again, this was a concern raised by her teacher, who suggested that Ellie may need to be seen by her general practitioner (GP) regarding her repeated sore throats. Following this discussion, Ellie's mum made an appointment to see the GP.

1   **In Ellie's case, how was the diagnosis and decision to treat through surgery reached?**

A   At several points during Ellie's consultation, which involved both her GP and then her ENT specialist.

Consultation with the GP

On examining Ellie, the GP found her to be pyrexic, with a temperature of 39.5°C. The lymph nodes in her neck appeared swollen, and her tonsils looked red and inflamed, with evidence of a slight halitosis (Cordbridge, 2011). Taking a detailed past medical history of Ellie's symptoms' from her mum, and reviewing his own clinical findings, he diagnosed recurrent tonsillitis: an inflammation of the tonsils usually caused by infection. The tonsils are glands composed of lymphatic tissue and are situated on each side of the oropharynx. They produce antibodies against infection and frequently serve as the site of acute infection (Smeltzer *et al.*, 2010: 599). The GP explained to both Ellie and her mum that he was going to refer her to see an ear, nose and throat (ENT) specialist, with a view to Ellie undergoing a tonsillectomy.

Consultation with the ENT specialist

Ellie and her mum went to see a consultant ENT surgeon, who on reading the GP's clinical referral letter, carried out a further clinical examination. The specialist's decision as to whether or not to operate depends largely on the history provided by the patient's GP (Milford and Rowlands, 1999). After discussing her own clinical findings with Ellie and her mum, the consultant explained that as Ellie had a high number of clinically significant and adequately treated sore throats in the preceding 12 months, causing her to miss a significant number of school days (SIGN, 2010), she felt it would be in the child's best health interests to schedule Ellie for a tonsillectomy.

According to the National Institute for Clinical Excellence (NICE, 2003), a tonsillectomy is given a grade 2 (intermediate) banding that suggests no preoperative tests – for example, chest x-ray, ECG or full blood count are required in a normally fit and healthy child like Ellie. Ellie's mum enquired whether or not the procedure could be carried out as a day surgery, as she felt that staying overnight in hospital would be too distressing for Ellie and, as she was a single mother, she had the care of her other child to consider. At least 90% of surgery in children can be performed as a day case (AAGBI, 2010). As Ellie was normally fit and well, and the consultant could appreciate the connection between mother and daughter and the impact Ellie's surgery would have on other family members, she agreed to the request and scheduled Ellie for a tonsillectomy as a day surgery patient.

Prior to Ellie's admittance to the day surgery unit, her mum received a letter detailing the date and time of her admission, the fasting time required and other relevant information regarding Ellie's admission. This was then followed up by a phone call to Ellie's home from the pre-admissions clinic to ascertain such information as previous medical or surgical history, allergies and dietary requirements. This process would be used to reduce the time taken to admit Ellie on the day of her tonsillectomy (Tanner, 2010).

2 **Can you describe how Ellie was admitted to the day case ward? Reflect on the various roles of those involved in Ellie's preoperative preparation.**

A On the day of Ellie's surgery, she and her mum arrived on the ward and were welcomed by her named nurse and the day surgery play therapist. Once Ellie was settled into a bed bay, her named nurse completed a set of baseline observations of Ellie's weight (30 kg), temperature (36.5°C), pulse (85 beats per minute), respiration (20 breaths per minute) and oxygen saturation (SpO_2) (98%). These baseline observations are within the normal parameters for a child of Ellie's age (Tanner, 2010).

Following the documentation of these observations, the role of the play therapist was explained to Ellie and her mum, and some of the activities available for Ellie to do while on the day surgery ward were demonstrated. The role of play therapists has proved particularly popular with both children and parents in the preparation of children undergoing general anaesthesia, and is reported to be of value in decreasing the anxiety associated with anaesthesia and surgery (O'Sullivan and Wong, 2013).

Ellie's named nurse introduced a doctor from the surgical team to Ellie and her mum. He was able to answer any questions they may have had regarding Ellie's procedure, and explained in more detail the benefits and risks involved with the surgical procedure – for example, postoperative bleeding and pain. Once full understanding and clarification had been sought by both parties, it was explained to Ellie and her mum that children under the age of 16 can consent to medical treatment if they have sufficient maturity and judgement to enable them fully to understand what is proposed (Cornock, 2007). Ellie requested that her mum sign the consent form on her behalf.

This was followed by a visit from the anaesthetist; the rationale for the preoperative visit is to ascertain from Ellie and her mum any past medical history that may have an effect on her anaesthetic care – for example, heart condition, recent cold or chest infection. The visit also enabled verbal consent from Ellie's mum to be given. A physical examination, which included listening to Ellie's chest to assess her respiratory function, was undertaken. The anaesthetist asked Ellie to open her mouth, to check for any loose teeth she may have. To assess her Mallampati classification, he asked her to put her tongue out as far as she could, to assess the possibility of difficulty with intubation or extubation (Carr and Harvey, 2003; Sundaram, 2003). The anaesthetist graded Ellie as a class 1 as he was able to visualise her soft palate, fauces, uvula and tonsillar pillars.

Stop and think

Ellie asked the anaesthetist if the needle would hurt as she was frightened of needles. What is the appropriate response?

Anxiety and agitation can markedly hinder the insertion of intravenous cannula (Litke, Pikulska and Wegner, 2012). The anaesthetist explained to Ellie that he would ask her named nurse to apply, in his words, some 'magic cream'. This contains tetracaine (Ametop), which was applied topically to the backs of Ellie's hands. Ametop gel can be applied over two areas with visible veins, e.g. on dorsal area of both hands. When Ametop gel is applied to the skin, the tetracaine prevents pain signals passing from that area to the brain and so numbs the skin. This means a needle can be inserted into a vein without causing pain (Litke *et al.*, 2012). In a study carried out involving 120 children undergoing cannulation, Arrowsmith (2000) compared the effectiveness of EMLA cream (eutectic mixture of local anaesthetics) and tetracaine (Ametop) gel in providing analgesia for venous cannulation. This study confirmed previous reports that Ametop gel rather than EMLA provides more effective topical anaesthesia prior to venous cannulation in a significantly higher proportion of children.

The anaesthetist also discussed with Ellie's mum the option of giving Ellie an inhalation anaesthetic through a clear face mask should Ellie still feel anxious in the anaesthetic room. The anaesthetist explained that he was more than happy for Ellie's mum to stay with her during the anaesthetic induction as this comforting presence can reduce the child's anxiety (Black and McEwan, 2004).

Prior to Ellie's procedure, the operating department practitioners (ODPs) prepared the perioperative environment to accommodate a child of Ellie's age to undergo a tonsillectomy procedure. The ODPs, as part of their role, prepared and checked the anaesthetic machine, breathing circuits, airway adjuncts and availability of required pharmacology. Similarly, an ODP working as a member of the scrubbed team prepared the required tonsillectomy set and undertook a count of all instrumentation, including the size 6 x 1 inch swabs that are routinely used for this type of surgery.

Other equipment – for example, the operating table and attachments, pressure-relieving gel pads, to include a gel-filled head ring to support Ellie's head, and a gel bag that was placed under her shoulder blades to assist with optimal surgical access, an electrosurgical bipolar diathermy machine used to control haemostasis and a surgical headlight to enable visualisation of Ellie's tonsils – were prepared and checked by the circulating ODP.

3 **Can you describe the range of anaesthetic equipment that should be available for Ellie's anaesthetic care?**

A Due to the nature of a tonsillectomy procedure and the potential risks – for example, the possibility of substantial bleeding – a regional or local anaesthetic is not a viable option for this type of surgery. Therefore a general anaesthetic was selected for Ellie's surgical procedure. During the team brief (WHO, 2008), the anaesthetist informed the ODP that, as Ellie was an average-size child, he wouldn't require a Miller paediatric straight-bladed laryngoscope. He was planning to intubate her using a Macintosh size 3 disposable laryngoscope blade to reduce risk of cross-infection, with a size 6.5 mm uncuffed pre-formed south-facing RAE tube positioned in the mid-line to provide good surgical access (Ravi and Howell, 2007).

Stop and think

How would you decide upon the appropriate size of endotracheal tube to use?

The formulae for gauging the correct size of endotracheal tube (ET) for a child of Ellie's age is to divide the child's age by 4 and then add 4 to the total (for example, Ellie is 10, so [10 ÷ 4] + 4 = 6.5). It is safe and best practice to have one size smaller and one size larger tube available. Consequently, a size 6.0 and 7.0 mm should also be available for use. As an alternative, a reinforced size 2.5 laryngeal mask airway (LMA) could also be considered for a tonsillectomy procedure. However, there are some disadvantages to using an LMA for this type of procedure as it doesn't offer the security of an endotracheal tube and can make surgical access difficult in small children (Ravi and Howell, 2007).

During an ear, nose and throat operation, the anaesthetic machine is positioned at the foot of the operating table to avoid any breakdown of the sterile surgical field and facilitate better surgical access. Therefore, the anaesthetist requested that a 2.4 m long Mapleson D classification Bain circuit with a 1-litre reservoir bag be attached to the anaesthetic machine. There are many advantages to using a breathing circuit of this type – for example, a valve is present at the proximal end to aid the control of the fresh gas that is always delivered at the patient end of the circuit, and to support the scavenging of waste anaesthetic gasses (Black and McEwan, 2004).

4 **List the drugs that would be required as part of Ellie's anaesthetic care.**

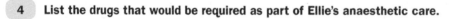

A To facilitate the administration of the intravenous pharmacological drugs, Ellie was can-nulated using a 22 g blue cannula. This would enable the administration of 2–5 mg/kg of propofol to induce anaesthesia. This is a fast-acting intravenous induction agent, which allows the stage of surgical anaesthesia to be achieved more rapidly than would the use of a gaseous induction (Morton, 1997). Studies have shown that propofol produces a lower incidence of postoperative nausea and vomiting (PONV) in children following tonsillectomy (Carr and Harvey, 2003). In addition, 1 mg/kg suxamethonium chloride was used to facilitate endotracheal intubation, with 150 μg/kg of dexameth-asone and 100 μg/kg of ondansetron to reduce the risk of PONV. Carr and Harvey (2003) suggest that children given ondansetron must be carefully observed postoper-atively following tonsillectomy as its actions may mask bleeding.

Pain following tonsillectomy is variable, with some children requiring postoperative opioid pain relief, such as 2 μg/kg fentanyl. Other children can be managed with a combination of a non-steroidal anti-inflammatory drug (NSAID) – for example, 12.5 mg diclofenac suppository inserted rectally prior to the surgical commencement, and paracetamol. Topical 1% lignocaine sprayed evenly over the tonsillar bed postoperatively has been shown to improve pain relief (Carr and Harvey, 2003).

Following induction, anaesthesia was then maintained with a combination of oxygen (O_2), nitrous oxide (N_2O) and sevoflurane. Standard monitoring in accordance with Association of Anaesthetists of Great Britain and Ireland (AAGBI) guidelines (AAGBI, 2007), to incorporate, ECG, BP, SaO_2 and $EtCO_2$ (capnography), was used throughout Ellie's surgical procedure.

As a tonsillectomy is a relatively short procedure, intermittent positive pressure ventilation (IPPV) was not required. Ellie did not therefore need a non-depolarising neuromuscular blocking drug such as atracurium. Consequently, the anaesthetist administered 30 mg of suxamethonium chloride, a depolarising neuromuscular blocking drug, to facilitate intubation. Following successful intubation with the 6.5 mm uncuffed, pre-formed south-facing RAE tube, and once spontaneous respiration was achieved, Ellie was transferred to the operating theatre.

5 **What specific positioning and instrumentation requirements are needed to perform a tonsillectomy?**

A Ellie was placed on to the operating table in a supine position. The anaesthetist and ODP carefully removed her pillow, ensuring not to dislodge the position of the ET tube, and exchanged it for a gel head ring. A gel pad was placed under her shoulders. These items are used to slightly extend the patient's neck and facilitate optimum surgical access. The circulating ODP opened the outer packaging of the tonsillectomy tray using a no-touch technique. In 2001, following a major health issue with Creutzfeldt-Jakob disease (CJD) and tonsillar surgery, the Department of Health (DH) recommended that reusable instruments should be discarded, with the aim that, by the end of 2001, usage of single-use instruments would be universally accepted. Studies revealed that the prion protein becomes positive in lymphoreticular tissue relatively early in the incubation period and, even if CJD has an incubation period of several decades, the impact of transmission to children through contaminated instruments was particularly serious (Frosh, Joyce and Johnson, 2001). However, due to concerns about the quality of the disposable instruments and complication rates, and more importantly patient safety, reusable instruments were reintroduced later that year (Sethi, Kane and Condon, 2013). The scrub ODP completed the instrument, swabs and needles count with the circulating ODP, and then assisted the surgeon with draping, first, Ellie's head in a surgical drape and then a larger drape was placed over her chest and abdomen to complete the sterile field. Prior to the commencement of surgery, the 'time out' pause was adhered to as part of the WHO Surgical Safety Checklist (WHO, 2008).

6 **Give a description of the surgical procedure and reflect upon your role as a scrubbed practitioner.**

A To commence the procedure, the surgeon placed a Boyle Davis gag into Ellie's mouth to retract her tongue and expose her oropharynx. The blade of the gag fits over the ET tube that the anaesthetist has positioned in the midline to provide good surgical access. As the gag is opened and held in place with the Drafton rods, it is important that the anaesthetist monitors the patient's $EtCO_2$ (capnography) as it is at this point that an occlusion of the ET tube could occur due to the Boyle Davis gag kinking the ET tube. Capnography provides further information in respect to adequacy of ventilation and other airway dynamics (Black and McEwan, 2004). Communication and teamwork between surgeon and anaesthetist are imperative during a shared airway procedure as they both require access to a remote area and must accommodate one another's requirements in care of the patient (Ravi and Howell, 2007).

To remove Ellie's tonsils, the surgeon used bipolar diathermy. This produces heat to dissect and incise the mucosa and divide the strands of tissue that bind the tonsils to the pharyngeal wall. The bipolar also aids haemostasis by coagulating any bleeding vessels (NICE, 2005). Haemorrhage is the most serious complication following tonsillectomy (Ravi and Howell, 2007); it is therefore imperative that the surgeon minimise bleeding. Using this bipolar technique means that no sutures or ties are required to support haemostasis. This is particularly advantageous with a day case procedure, as it shortens the operation time.

Bleeding post-tonsillectomy can occur within the first 24 hours (primary haemorrhage) or after 24 hours (secondary haemorrhage). This can lead to some patients being readmitted to undergo further surgery (NICE, 2005). A large clot, sometimes called a 'coroner's clot', can be left in the post nasal space (PNS) following tonsillectomy. If undetected, it could easily be inhaled into the trachea and block the child's airway (Hatfield and Tronson, 2014). With this in mind, the surgeon used a dental mirror to visualise Ellie's PNS at the end of the procedure and this was clear of any blood clots.

Once the procedure was complete, the instruments, swabs and needles were counted for the final time to ensure that the count was complete prior to Ellie leaving the operating theatre.

7   **What must be considered when Ellie is extubated at the end of her surgery?**

A   The dilemma of whether to extubate the patient when fully awake and able to protect their own airway, or still deeply anaesthetised to avoid a 'stormy' emergence and bleeding, will always exist following a tonsillectomy procedure (Ravi and Howell, 2007). Following Ellie's procedure, her anaesthetist decided to extubate the child while she was still deeply anaesthetised so as not to risk her coughing and causing any unnecessary bleeding. Therefore, the child was turned on to her left side and a pillow was placed under her hips to tilt her slightly head down. This position would allow any blood to drain from the child's mouth (Hatfield and Tronson, 2014). Following extubation, the ODP placed a suitably sized face mask over Ellie's mouth. The mask and tubing were connected to an O_2 cylinder under the patient's trolley and the flow meter on the cylinder was adjusted to administer 4 litres per minute of oxygen.

Ellie was then prepared for transfer to the post-anaesthetic care unit (PACU), where her care was handed over to the PACU ODPs.

8   **How is the PACU prepared to receive Ellie?**

A   Prior to Ellie being transferred to the PACU, the ODP prepared the environment to receive a child who had undergone a tonsillectomy procedure. This would include: pipeline O_2 supply with cylinder back-up, and a Bain circuit suitable for spontaneous and controlled ventilation (Black and McEwan, 2004). A range of uncuffed ET tubes, LMAs and other airway adjuncts would also be available. Suction apparatus, with a selection of soft catheters, would also be made available.

q Can you list the range of assessments required to ensure Ellie's optimum postoperative recovery?

A On arriving into the PACU, the ABCDE patient assessment protocol was followed and Ellie was connected to the piped O_2 supply. ECG, BP and SpO_2 recordings were monitored and documented in her care plan. In line with the core approaches to pain assessment for children identified by Carter and Jonas (2010), the ODP was constantly carrying out a physiological assessment, checking Ellie's colour, respiratory rate and observing any behavioural changes that may indicate an expression of pain. Signs of excessive swallowing should be noted, as this may be a symptom of bleeding in the back of her throat. Ellie regained consciousness, and began to cry and ask for her mum.

Prior to 2013 the opioid of choice for a child of Ellie's age having undergone a tonsillectomy procedure would have been codeine. However, due to three reported cases of child deaths after being administered codeine, the Medicines and Healthcare Products Regulatory Agency issued advice (MHPRA, 2013) that codeine should be used only in children over 12 years old. Therefore, Ellie was prescribed Oramorph elixir 0.2–0.4 mg/kg, oral paracetamol 20 mg/kg and a stat dose of 10 mg/kg of ibuprofen.

Ellie told the ODP that she felt like she wanted to be sick. Again, the ODP re-assured Ellie, offering her emotional support. Ellie had already received dexamethasone, so in order to adopt a multimodal approach she was further prescribed ondansetron; this acts as an antagonist of $5\text{-}HT_3$ receptor in the vomiting centre of the brain to potentiate the action of the dexamethasone (Hanisch, 2010). The ODP explained that the sickness feeling would soon pass and she would ask for Ellie's mum to be brought to the PACU to comfort her. Litke *et al.* (2012) found that it was extremely important that a parent is present in the PACU to support their child's recovery from anaesthesia.

When Ellie had met the PACU discharge criteria, the PACU ODP gave a thorough handover to the ward nurse outlining the main details of the surgical procedure. This handover should establish thoroughly the child's current physical status before discharging Ellie from the PACU back to the ward (Hatfield and Tronson, 2014).

10 What are the care considerations for Ellie following her discharge from the day surgery unit?

A Following her tonsillectomy, Ellie experienced a painful throat for approximately five to seven days, during which time this was alleviated by ibuprofen and paracetamol. She was encouraged to eat solid foods and drink plenty of water to help her throat heal. She was given two weeks off school to aid her recovery and reduce the risk of picking up any infections from her classmates (NHS, 2013).

11 Can you begin to reflect holistically on Ellie's experience and the multidisciplinary approach to her care?

A A holistic approach was adopted throughout this child's experience. This was evident following the first meeting between her teacher and her mum. The teacher was concerned that as Ellie wasn't eating normally and also missing a number of days from school, there may have been some social or domestic reason behind the child's behaviour. The family GP was very supportive towards Ellie and her mum, recognising the need for an early surgical intervention due to the discomfort the child was experiencing and the impact it was having on her schooling. The roles that Ellie's named nurse and the play therapist took in this case were paramount to her overall care. They were able to support her emotional state not only by building a rapport with both Ellie and her mum when they entered the ward, but also by engaging her with activities to keep her mind active while she was on the ward.

The care and support Ellie and her mum received from the theatre team was holistic in its approach and designed to meet their individual requirements. During the preoperative visit, both the surgeon and the anaesthetist were more than happy to answer any questions and relieve any anxiety that was expressed by Ellie or her mum. On entering the PACU, the ODP caring for Ellie demonstrated an understanding of her emotional status as well as being aware of her physical requirements. Overall, the experience that Ellie and her mum have had during this case study highlights that each patient should be treated as an individual and, ultimately, we as practitioners must remember to always consider the patient as a person and not just a surgical procedure.

REFERENCES AND FURTHER READING

Arrowsmith, J. (2000) A comparison of local anaesthetics for venipuncture. *Archives of Disease in Childhood,* **82**: 309–310.

Association of Anaesthetists of Great Britain and Ireland (AAGBI) (2007) *Recommendations for Standards of Monitoring During Anaesthesia and Recovery.* London: AAGBI.

Association of Anaesthetists of Great Britain and Ireland (AAGBI) (2010) *Pre-operative Assessment and Patient Preparation: The Role of the Anaesthetist.* London: AAGBI.

Black, A. and McEwan, A. (2004) *Paediatric and Neonatal Anaesthesia: Anaesthesia in a Nutshell.* Edinburgh: Butterworth Heinemann.

British and Irish Legal Information Institute (1985) Gillick v. West Norfolk and Wisbech Area Health Authority. Available online at: www.bailii.org/uk/cases/UKHL/1985/7.html (accessed 8 July 2014).

Carr, A. and Harvey, A. (2003) Anaesthesia principles and techniques, in Morton, N. and Peutrell, J. (eds) *Paediatric Anaesthesia and Critical Care in the District Hospital.* Edinburgh: Butterworth Heinemann.

Carter, B. and Jonas, D. (2010) Nursing care and management of children's perioperative pain, in Shields, L. (ed.) *Perioperative Care of a Child: A Nursing Manual.* Oxford: Wiley Blackwell.

Cordbridge, R. (2011) *Essential ENT* (2nd edn). London: Hodder Arnold.

Cornock, M. (2007) Fraser guidelines or Gillick competence? *Journal of Children's and Young People's Nursing,* **1**(3): 142.

Frosh, A., Joyce, R. and Johnson, A. (2001) Iatrogenic vCJD from surgical instruments. *British Medical Journal,* **322**(7302): 1558–1559.

Hanisch, E. (2010) The paediatric post-anaesthetic care unit, in Shields, L. (ed.) *Perioperative Care of a Child: A Nursing Manual.* Oxford: Wiley Blackwell.

Hatfield, A. and Tronson, M. (2014) *The Complete Recovery Room Book* (5th edn). Oxford: Oxford University Press.

Litke, J., Pikulska, A. and Wegner, T. (2012) Management of perioperative stress in children and parents. *Anaesthesiology Intensive Therapy*, **44**(3): 170–174.

Medicines and Healthcare Products Regulatory Agency (MHPRA) (2013) Codeine for analgesia: restricted use in children because of reports of morphine toxicity. *Drug Safety Update*, **6**(12): 1–2.

Milford, C. and Rowlands, A. (1999) *Shared Care for ENT*. Oxford: Isis Medical Media.

Morton, N.S. (1997) *Assisting the Anaesthetist*. Oxford: Oxford University Press.

National Institute for Clinical Excellence (NICE) (2003) Preoperative tests: the use of preoperative tests for elective surgery. Available online at: www.nice.org.uk/guidance/cg3 (accessed 10 March 2014).

National Institute for Health and Clinical Excellence (NICE) (2005) Electrosurgery (diathermy and coblation) for tonsillectomy. Available online at: www.nice.org.uk/guidance/ipg150/chapter/2-the-procedure (accessed 17 March 2014).

NHS (2013) Treating tonsillitis. Available online at: www.nhs.uk/Conditions/Tonsllitis (accessed 18 March 2014).

O'Sullivan, M. and Wong, G.K. (2013) Preinduction techniques to relieve anxiety in children undergoing general anaesthesia. *Continuing Education in Anaesthesia, Critical Care and Pain*, **13**(6): 196–199.

Ravi, R. and Howell, T. (2007) Anaesthesia for paediatric ear, nose and throat surgery. *Continuing Education in Anaesthesia, Critical Care and Pain*, **7**(2): 33–37.

Royal College of Surgeons (RCS) (2013) Tonsillectomy commissioning guide. Available online at: www.rcseng.ac.uk/healthcare-bodies/docs/published-guides/tonsillectomy (accessed 11 March 2014).

Sethi, N., Kane, J. and Condon, L. (2013) Creutzfeldt-Jakob disease and ENT. *Journal of Laryngology and Otology*, **127**: 1050–1055.

SIGN (2010) Management of sore throat and indications for tonsillectomy: a national clinical guideline. Available online at: www.sign.ac.uk (accessed 7 March 2014).

Smeltzer, S., Bare, B., Hinkle, J. and Cheever, K. (2010) *Brunner and Suddarth's Textbook of Medical-Surgical Nursing* (12th edn). Philadelphia: Lippincott Williams & Wilkins.

Sundaram, R. (2003) Predicting difficult intubation: useful or what? A response to 'Predicting difficult intubation – worthwhile exercise or pointless ritual?' *Anaesthesia*, **57**: 105–109.

Tanner, A. (2010) Day surgery for children, in Shields, L. (ed.) *Perioperative Care of a Child: A Nursing Manual*. Oxford: Wiley Blackwell.

World Health Organization (WHO) (2008) WHO Surgical Safety Checklist. Available online at: www.who.int/patientsafety/safesurgery/tools_resources/SSSL_Checklist_finalJun08.pdf (accessed 17 March 2014).

Vaginal hysterectomy: the care of Anelia Woods

Kelly Goffin

INTRODUCTION AND LEARNING OUTCOMES

This case study details the perioperative care of a female patient undergoing a hysterectomy. This procedure is the most frequently performed surgical procedure within the specialism (McCracken and Lefebvre, 2007). Vaginal hysterectomy is the removal of the uterus and cervix through the vagina, and is the preferred method for benign gynaecological conditions. Stovall and Mann (2015) argue that vaginal hysterectomy holds fewer complications and is associated with a shorter hospital stay, along with a faster postoperative recovery time.

By the end of this case study you will be able to:

- discuss the specific issues surrounding the holistic care of a patient undergoing vaginal hysterectomy following a prolapsed uterus
- identify and explain the preoperative preparation, anaesthetic care and surgical care of a patient undergoing a vaginal hysterectomy
- describe the surgical technique, alongside the intraoperative care and the subsequent post-anaesthetic recovery associated with vaginal hysterectomy.

Case outline

Anelia Woods is a 61-year-old female who is post-menopausal and presented to the gynaecological outpatient clinic with a six-month history of a prolapsed uterus. During her appointment with the gynaecologist a vaginal examination was performed and a second-degree prolapsed uterus diagnosed. The option of having a vaginal hysterectomy was offered to her as treatment of her presenting symptoms.

The possibility of an operative treatment comes as a relief to Anelia, as over the past six months her quality of life has been significantly affected through pain and constant worry of being unable participate in her hobbies, such as gardening; she is however also feeling slightly anxious at the prospect of an operation, especially to remove a part of her body that she feels 'makes her a woman'. She also has a number of 'practical' matters to consider, such as who will take care of the home and her husband while she is in hospital recovering from her surgery.

While in the clinic Anelia's baseline observations were recorded to ascertain if she was fit enough to undergo the proposed procedure. Her blood pressure was 132/80 mmHg, she had a regular pulse of 72 bpm and oxygen saturations of 98% were noted. Her weight of 62 kg was within normal range for her height, as her BMI is 24. No significant past medical history was noted. Anelia has had two children via vaginal delivery with no complications. This is important to consider; had Anelia delivered her children via Caesarean section there may be abdominal adhesions, which could make the procedure more complicated. The only regular medication she is currently taking is hormone replacement therapy (HRT) and she has no known allergies. Anelia is taking HRT in the form of Livial (tibolone) 2.5 mg once a day to improve her quality of life due to the symptoms she experiences associated with menopause, including hot flushes, vaginal dryness and sleep problems.

Stop and think

How might the concerns for her home and the care of her husband impact on Anelia's preparation for surgery?

1 **Prior to surgery, what support could be put in place to help Anelia understand her anxiety about the emotional impact of undergoing a hysterectomy?**

A Apart from providing ongoing emotional support in the operating theatre, prior to surgery a range of health professionals, including ODPs, should take time to help patients understand their anxieties and fears. Because this type of surgery is considered to be elective there can be a tendency for staff to view it as mundane and routine. However, for the patient this is not the case and they should be offered as much information and choice as possible.

Hysterectomy can lead to altered feelings of sexuality that may occur for a variety of physiological and psychological reasons. Symptoms that necessitate a hysterectomy can impact upon a couple's intimacy, which can continue after surgery. Some women may have experienced prolonged periods of pain and discomfort for many years, such that they may continue to avoid any sexual activity postoperatively. For other women, surgery can lead to a heightened sense of sexual responsiveness, which may have previously been repressed. As a patient support group, the Hysterectomy Association (2015) points to the fact that, in its view, there is a link between the amount of information provided and the greater perception of being cared for. Furthermore, it is claimed that providing the patient with as much information as possible around the procedure, and its risks and benefits, can lead to reduced postoperative complications.

Involvement of the sexual partner in the patient's care and treatment can also provide a greater degree of emotional support. A lack of understanding of the nature of female anatomy can lead to misunderstandings around sexuality postoperatively as both women and men can feel that hysterectomy has a negative effect on libido and on feelings of femininity. Alternatively, male indifference to surgical removal of the uterus could result from their own personal feelings of anxiety and guilt about acts of future sexual intimacy. However, it is interesting to note that, although counselling services are routinely offered to patients experiencing fertility treatment, this is not the case in respect of patients undergoing hysterectomy.

2   **What preparation was required prior to Anelia's surgery?**

A   Anelia's preoperative preparation consisted of a range routine blood tests, including full blood count. Within normal range preoperative haemoglobin levels of 13.5 g/dl were also recorded, along with a 12-lead ECG to ascertain the likelihood of any cardiac complications.

Consent to proceed with the procedure was also taken and time was given to explaining to Anelia the risks and benefits of vaginal hysterectomy so that she could make an informed choice about whether or not to go ahead with the surgery. The benefits were explained to her, namely improvement in and relief from her symptoms. The risks and associated complications from the surgery were explained, those being primarily associated with infection and postoperative bleeding, with also a greater risk of bladder injury caused as a direct result of the surgery (Clarke-Pearson and Geller, 2013).

Anelia may also benefit from some preoperative counselling to help her with her apprehensions of how she may feel from having her uterus removed, and how she perceives this will affect her femininity.

In this case, preparing the theatre for a vaginal hysterectomy included the preparation of an appropriate operating table capable of placing the patient into a lithotomy position. Allen legs, or lithotomy poles, to place Anelia in the correct position to optimise surgical access were required. The surgical team also prepared all the surgical equipment, including ensuring the availability of colporrhaphy surgical instruments, and diathermy to aid in intraoperative haemostasis. The availability of mobile theatre lights should also be ensured, in order to facilitate a more effective shadowless field for surgery.

3   **Describe the most appropriate anaesthetic technique, and consider which drugs could be administered as part of this anaesthetic.**

A   On arrival to the anaesthetic room a number of checks should be completed, adhering at all times to the WHO Surgical Safety Checklist. Anelia has no known allergies and no metal prosthetics or implants within her body; she does however have a crown on her top teeth. Being aware of any metal prosthetics is an important aspect to consider in relation to the use of monopolar diathermy, which will potentially be used during the procedure to seal blood vessels and limit the amount of blood loss experienced. The current from the diathermy enters the patient through the small-area active electrode and exits safely through the large-area return electrode via a diathermy plate (Sudhindra et al., 2000) – if the plate is incorrectly positioned this could lead to diathermy-related injuries. The application of routine anaesthetic monitoring should be explained to the patient in an attempt to reduce patient anxiety, which is raised following the application of monitoring.

Anelia had chosen to have a spinal anaesthetic with additional sedation, having previously expressed a wish not to be aware of what was happening to her within the operating theatre given her state of anxiety. Anelia was positioned for the spinal anaesthetic in a sitting-up position, slightly bent forward to expose her back. The ODP and perioperative support worker stayed in close contact with Anelia, both to help her maintain the correct position to facilitate the introduction of the spinal, and to help support, reassure and encourage her.

Diamorphine was included with Marcain® in the spinal anaesthetic, and additional sedation was also provided using propofol, which is an induction agent used for the induction and maintenance of anaesthetic, as well as maintenance of intraoperative light sedation, usually administered via a syringe pump. In Anelia's case, IV antibiotics such as metronidazole will also be required to prevent the risk of postoperative infection. Alternatively, a general anaesthetic could have been offered, however the risk of postoperative nausea and vomiting (PONV) and other negative effects such as a sore throat caused from the insertion of airway devices, combined with reduced opportunities for postoperative pain control, led Anelia to choose a spinal anaesthetic.

4 **How was Anelia prepared for surgery? You should consider the measures taken to minimise the risk of harm.**

A Patient positioning is of the utmost importance. This aspect of surgical care can carry many potential risks, which can cause unnecessary harm. When using the lithotomy position it is especially important to ensure that all bony prominences are protected, such as the sacral area and elbows; standard pressure area care should be adopted by placing gel pads under the affected parts. Nerve damage can also occur such that particular attention should be given to the lateral aspect of the calf; this will ensure that excessive pressure should not lead to a compression injury to the perineal nerve (Lucero and Shah, 2010). Femoral nerve damage can also occur due to the suspension of the legs in this position because of excessive abduction to the legs. Anelia's buttocks should be placed as close to the edge of the operating table as possible, to ensure ease of access for the placement of retractors to aid surgical access.

A diathermy plate should also be sited in a clean, hairless area to ensure sufficient contact is maintained between the patient and the plate. In Anelia's case the abdomen was selected as a suitable place for the plate to be positioned in. Because the lithotomy position requires the patient's legs to be placed in a raised position, this could affect the placement and contact of the plate due to poor adhesion. Understanding the nature of the procedure, Anelia had already removed any excess hair from her pubic region prior to being admitted for surgery.

In Anelia's case Savlon solution (chlorhexidine gluconate with cetrimide) was used for the surgical preparation of the vagina and surrounding area. Immediately prior to the start of the procedure, Anelia was draped using a pair of lithotomy leggings, a medium drape, which was placed under the buttocks to cover the colporrhaphy table, and another to cover the abdomen to ensure a sterile surgical field was clearly delineated and maintained. A 12 ch Foley catheter with 10 ml sterile water to inflate the balloon was inserted into Anelia's bladder and a standard catheter bag attached. Catheterisation is used to help monitor urine output and to observe any colour changes (due to the presence of blood) to her urine, which may indicate injury or perforation to her bladder or ureter. It should also be noted that, due to the effects of the spinal anaesthetic, Anelia will be unable to feel the need to urinate on her own until the spinal begins to wear off.

Anelia's body temperature was monitored and maintained throughout the procedure by an upper torso warming blanket connected to a forced air warming device such as a 'Bair Hugger'. Maintenance of normal temperature ranges is important to minimise the increased rate of wound infection, pressure sores, and also a longer stay in both recovery and hospital (Harper, Andrzejowski and Alexander, 2008).

Although minimal blood loss was anticipated, additional intraoperative fluids were administered via 1 litre of Hartmann's solution (a crystalloid solution) to mitigate against the hypotension resulting from spinal anaesthesia. It should be noted that colloid solutions were also available if required as these contain large molecules and are designed to remain in the intravenous space longer than crystalloid fluids, to the degree that colloids are better than crystalloids at expanding the circulatory volume. This is because their larger molecules are retained more easily in the intravascular space (Kwan, Bunn and Roberts, 2003).

5   **Describe a typical surgical technique necessary to perform a vaginal hysterectomy.**

A   The following vaginal hysterectomy surgical technique is adapted from Lucero and Shah (2010), and Stark, Gerli and di Renzo (2006).

- A weighted speculum is placed into the vagina, the cervix is then secured with two Teale Vulsellums and traction is applied. Next, a solution of local anaesthetic is injected sub-mucosally, which contains 80 ml sodium chloride (NaCl) mixed with 0.25% bupivacaine with adrenaline 1:200,000. This acts as a vasoconstrictor for the purpose of hydro-dissection and haemostasis.
- Initial incision of the vaginal wall is made with a blade around the cervix, the bladder is then detached and separated from the uterus by being pushed upwards; bladder injury occurs in 2% of vaginal hysterectomies (Maresh *et al.*, 2002). The anterior peritoneum is then exposed, and a retractor inserted to keep the bladder out of the way and to protect from any damage. The posterior peritoneum is subsequently exposed, including the pouch of Douglas.
- The vaginal pedicles are now ready to be excised and sutured. First the sacrouterine ligaments are clamped, dissected and ligated with these pedicles, leaving the suture long for identification purposes and with a Dunhill clamp secured to the drapes. Next the cardinal ligaments are clamped bilaterally with a curved Maingot clamp, dissected and then ligated securely. At this point, the ureter should be identified, as it is essential to ensure that no damage has occurred.

Next the uterine vessels and broad ligaments, including peritoneum, are clamped to minimise bleeding from pedicles. The round ligament and ovarian ligaments, and associated blood vessels, are next and are secured with one free tie and a second transfixion suture. The uterus can now be removed and should be inspected on either side; the pedicles should be inspected for bleeding prior to closing the vaginal vault. A swab on a stick is available to push the bowel out of the way so as not to damage it and the vault is sutured continuously starting at the angles of the vault.

In Anelia's case wound closure was carried out using 0 Vicryl to secure the abdominal muscle layer and 2/0 Vicryl Rapide was selected for subcutaneous skin closure, but this was largely done to the surgeon's preference. The vagina was packed with a gauze pack to help with haemostasis. Due to a lack of oestrogen caused by the menopause in Anelia's case, the pack was soaked in Ortho-Gynest cream. A sanitary towel was also used in case of any postoperative vaginal discharge or bleeding. No wound drainage was required.

Stop and think

What type of specific surgical instrumentation is needed to perform a vaginal hysterectomy?

A gynaecological repair tray was selected, which specifically included the following:

- two Teale Vulsellums (a weighted vaginal retractor)
- curved and straight clamps, such as Maingots, Gwilliams, Howkins, Spencer Wells and straight Dunhills
- specific lateral wall retractors to improve access, such as Landons
- a size 10 blade on a No. 3 BP handle; a pair of Gillies and/or Lanes dissecting forceps
- heavy curved mayo scissors and straight mayo scissors
- monopolar diathermy forceps, used to assist in haemostasis.

---

6 **Explore the specific care that Anelia received in the post-anaesthetic care unit (PACU) and during her longer-term recovery.**

(A) There were no specific transfer requirements needed from the operating theatre to the recovery area. On arrival, following a handover from the anaesthetist and scrub practitioner, responsibility transferred to the recovery practitioner. Patient assessment within the PACU should focus on both the recovery from spinal anaesthesia (return of sensation) and the surgery itself.

Any postoperative bleeding was observed and recorded. Urine output was monitored and checked for the presence of blood in the urine, which could indicate bladder trauma during the procedure. Low urine outputs could indicate possible damage to either of the ureters during surgery. In Anelia's case, discharge from the PACU occurred when the recovery practitioner was satisfied that she was comfortable and stable enough to be returned to the care of the ward staff. Postoperatively the vaginal pack was removed after 24 hours, along with the urinary catheter, although Anelia was monitored closely for a further period of time until she passed urine, to check that she was not at risk of urinary retention.

Anelia's long-term recovery begins with regular pain relief, such as a non-steroidal anti-inflammatory drug (NSAID), such as diclofenac or ibuprofen. If constipation is experienced this should be treated with a daily dose of lactulose. After discharge from hospital Anelia was advised to avoid heavy lifting and strenuous exercise for a minimum of three months, although driving could be commenced six weeks postoperatively at the point that an emergency stop could be performed safely without physical discomfort. Rest and exercise are important factors in the longer-term recovery from a vaginal hysterectomy. A slight vaginal discharge is normally experienced for a few weeks following surgery, and Anelia was advised to seek medical advice if this became offensive, bright red or heavy with clots.

7   **Are there any specific cultural aspects of hysterectomy that need to be considered?**

A   Time and understanding should be given to let women explore their feelings and emotional response to having a hysterectomy, and in this respect healthcare professionals can act as a source of comfort (Corney et al., 1992). As the womb is viewed as the core of womanhood many women may find it difficult to come to terms with the end of their fertility; indeed some cultures may find this operation particularly hard to accept. Roy (2004) asserts that there is little doubt that, for many women, loss of their uterus leads to feelings of grief. West Indian women see menstruation as a cleansing act, ridding the body of impurities. Some also fear they will be 'less of a woman' in the eyes of male partners. The cultural role of Muslim women can be dependent on their fertility, and again it may be difficult for both partners to come to terms with this following surgery.

REFERENCES AND FURTHER READING

Clarke-Pearson, D.L. and Geller, E.J. (2013) Complications of hysterectomy. *Obstetrics and Gynaecology*, **121**(3): 654–673.

Corney, R., Everett, H., Howells, A. and Crowther, M. (1992) The care of patients undergoing surgery for gynaecological cancer: the need for information, emotional support and counseling. *Journal of Advanced Nursing*, **17**(6): 667–671.

Harper, C.M., Andrzejowski, J.C. and Alexander, R. (2008) Editorial II: NICE and warm. *British Journal of Anaesthesia*, **101**(3): 293–295.

Hysterectomy Association (2015) The emotional impact of hysterectomy. Available online at: www.hysterectomy-association.org.uk/information/the-emotional-impact-of-hysterectomy (accessed 27 October 2014).

Kwan, I., Bunn, F. and Roberts, I. (2003) Timing and volume of fluid administration for patients with bleeding following trauma. *Cochrane Database of Systematic Reviews*, 3: CD002245.

Lucero, M. and Shah, A.D. (2010) Vaginal hysterectomy for the prolapsed uterus. *Clinical Obstetrics and Gynecology*, **53**(1): 26–39.

Maresh, M.J., Metcalfe, M.A., McPherson, K., Overton, C., Hall, V., Hargreaves, J., Bridgman, S., Dobbins, J. and Casbard, A. (2002) The VALUE national hysterectomy study: description of the patients and their surgery. *BJOG: An International Journal of Obstetrics and Gynaecology*, **109**: 302–312.

McCracken, M.B. and Lefebvre, G.G. (2007) Vaginal hysterectomy: dispelling the myths. *Journal of Obstetrics and Gynaecology*, **29**(5): 424–428.

Roy, R. (2004) *Chronic Pain, Loss and Suffering*. Toronto: University of Toronto Press.

Stark, M., Gerli, S. and di Renzo, G.C. (2006) An example for an optimised technique: the ten-step vaginal hysterectomy. *Progress in Obstetrics and Gynecology*, **17**: 358–368.

Stovall, T.G. and Mann, W.J. (2015) Patient information: vaginal hysterectomy. Available online at: www.uptodate.com/contents/vaginal-hyaterectomy-beyond-the-basics (accessed 11 September 2015).

Sudhindra, T.V., Joseph, A., Hacking, C.J. and Haray, P.N. (2000) Are surgeons aware of the dangers of diathermy? *Annals of the Royal College of Surgeons of England*, **82**: 31–32.

PART 2
Suggested 2nd Year (Level 5) Case Studies

Bilateral mastectomy: the care of Louise Mullaney

Agnes Lafferty

INTRODUCTION AND LEARNING OUTCOMES

This case study details the perioperative care of a young female undergoing prophy-lactic bilateral mastectomies. Genetic testing had indicated that she had BRCA2 genetic mutation that increased her lifetime risk of developing breast cancer. Hoskins and Greene (2012) state that the 'cumulative lifetime risks' of the development of breast cancer for BRCA1 or BRCA2 carriers are between 50% and 85%.

By the end of this case study you will be able to:

- explain the care needs of and the practical issues considered by BRCA1 or BRCA2 genetic mutation positive patients
- consider the perioperative management of women presenting for prophylactic mastectomy
- discuss the surgical reconstructive techniques available for women undergoing prophylactic mastectomy.

Case outline

Louise Mullaney is a 33-year-old married female with two children. She has a mutation in the gene BRCA2 and has a strong family history of cancer. BRCA genes 1 and 2 block the inappropriate development and division of cells. Muta-tions in these genes can, therefore, enable cells to proliferate unchecked and consequently develop into tumours (Smith, 2012).

Her eldest child, a girl, is three years old and her youngest child, a boy, is aged one. She recently stopped breastfeeding her son and has decided that her family is complete. Louise's maternal aunts suffered breast and ovarian cancer. Her mother underwent surgery for breast cancer, and was subsequently tested and found to have mutation in the BRCA2 gene. Her mother is currently well with no diagnosed metastatic disease. Her older sister, Marie, died at age 28 from metastatic bowel cancer, having been genetically predisposed to bowel cancer and having had extensive surgery. Marie's two children are currently being cared for by Louise's mother.

Louise and her younger sister, Deborah, were tested and Louise was found to have mutation in the BRCA2 gene, while her sister was identified as being genetically at risk of developing bowel cancer. Louise was 32 weeks pregnant when tested. She decided to defer surgery until she had breastfed her son and was definitely sure that her family was complete.

Louise's husband, although anxious, was very supportive of her decisions. Hoskins and Greene (2012) found that partners of young BRCA-positive women can become very involved in decision making and planning for management of the risk of developing breast cancer. Louise also reported a heavy reliance on her family. This mirrors phenomena reported by Samson *et al.* (2014), who found that women living with the BRCA1 and BRCA2 mutations drew support mainly from inner social circles such as family, husbands and close friends. Louise underwent preoperative counselling before making her decision to have surgery. She maintained, however, that her strong family support and her exposure to such extensive experience of illness and surgery informed her decisions. She felt that her decision to have elective bilateral prophylactic mastectomies with reconstructions was right for her.

Stop and think

Think about how you would care for Louise. What do you think are her main concerns and anxieties around both her decisions, and the impact of these upon her surgery and her recovery, including her physical and emotional well-being, including body image (and intimacy).

1 **Prior to surgery Louise attended counselling. What was the counsellor's role and how did this contribute to Louise's care?**

A The purpose of the counselling was to explore the issues that might affect her reaction to the news that she had the BRCA2 mutation and consequent increased risk of developing breast and ovarian cancer.

Louise's counsellor was convinced that Louise was well informed and displayed a good understanding of her management options and the implications of surgery. Hoskins and Greene (2012) indicate that the options available to BRCA-positive women with regard to managing the risk of breast cancer are surveillance, chemotherapeutic options and risk-reducing surgery. Louise was adamant that the most appropriate option for her was prophylactic mastectomies, as informed by the recent death of her sister and her experience of her mother's breast surgery.

Louise was also counselled by a breast care specialist nurse, to support her to make decisions that were most appropriate for her. Benedet (2011) champions the role of the specialist breast nurse in the UK as the provider of psychological care, information and practical advice to patients and their significant others throughout the process of care for breast cancer. Benedet (2011) further holds that breast cancer specialist nurses are pivotal in assessing the patient's anxiety levels, and emotional and sexual well-being, as well as acting as the conduit for referral to appropriate practitioners.

2 **A range of surgical treatment options may have been available to Louise. Can you list as many of these as possible and consider both the advantages and disadvantages of each?**

A When you have answered the above question, review the suggested options below and consider if you think Louise made the right choice and why?

Mastectomies with or without nipple sparing

Patients have the choice of mastectomies with or without nipple sparing. Sparing the nipple provides residual sensory function. Mastectomies without nipple sparing result in a loss of normal sensation. Kurian and Ford (2011) argue that there is insufficient data to compare the efficacy of nipple-sparing techniques with those where more breast tissue is removed. Niemeyer *et al.* (2011) and Nestle-Kramling and Kühn (2012), however, argue that nipple-sparing mastectomy is a safe prophylactic procedure. Louise was determined to maximise the amount of breast tissue removed to try to reduce her subsequent risk of developing breast cancer and therefore decided against nipple-sparing procedures. Other patients, however, may opt for nipple-sparing prophylactic mastectomies to maintain sensory function following surgery.

Breast reconstruction with implants

Breast reconstruction using implants can be carried out as a one- or two-stage procedure. In a one-stage technique, enough skin must be available to accommodate the implant. Louise had small breasts and consequently this procedure was not suitable. A two-stage technique requires tissue expanders to be inserted under the pectoral muscles. Inflation ports are placed under the skin of the chest or underarm. Following wound healing, the tissue expanders are inflated by injecting saline at one- to two-week intervals, stretching the chest wall tissue. These injections continue until the tissue expander is slightly larger than required. This helps the new breast achieve a more natural droop. Once the tissue expander is inflated to the required size, the saline is left in place to enable the skin to stretch. Finally, the tissue expander is replaced with a permanent silicone implant. The process of inflation can cause discomfort, tightness and pain over the breast area for up to 48 hours post-inflation (Cancer Research UK, 2012b; DellaCroce and Wolfe, 2013).

Louise opted for this technique because she was thin and wanted to have as much breast tissue and skin removed as possible with the perceived aim of minimising her subsequent risk of developing breast cancer. Nestle-Kramling and Kühn (2012) state, however, that skin and nipple-sparing techniques are accepted as safe and provide optimal aesthetic results. Nevertheless, Louise was keen to minimise her operation and recovery time so she could return to caring for her children as soon as possible. Macmillan Cancer Support (2014) advise that the two-stage technique is suitable for women undergoing bilateral procedures and who have small breasts as it gives good aesthetic results and involves a relatively short operating time compared to autogenous breast reconstruction (see below). DellaCroce and Wolfe (2013) also advise that implant reconstruction techniques have shorter recovery times with no donor site morbidity, are technically easier and are therefore more widely available than flap procedures.

Limitations, however, are mainly aesthetic and include a look that is less natural. The prosthetic breasts are not as soft or warm as natural breasts and achieve a less natural shape. They are usually higher than natural breasts and the prostheses can give rise to a 'rippling' effect in the skin. Complications can include bleeding and pain. Antibiotics are prescribed to minimise the risk of infection, which can occur in up to 10% of procedures. Similarly, one in ten women experience capsular contracture (Macmillan Cancer Support, 2014) caused by tightening of scar tissue around the implant making it the most common complication following breast reconstruction using implants (Medicines and Healthcare Products Regulatory Agency, 2012; Petit *et al.*, 2012).

Autogenous breast reconstruction

This technique uses the patient's own tissue to create new 'breast' tissue. The benefits are largely aesthetic given that the shape and droop are more natural than achieved with implants. Limitations, however, include the addition of donor site scars and the drawback that transplanted tissue may be a different colour from natural breast tissue. Furthermore, autogenous breast reconstruction procedures involve longer operating times, longer recovery times and longer hospitalisation (Sweetland, 2006). There are, however, several types of autogenous breast reconstruction, as described below.

- Latissimus dorsi flap in which the latissimus dorsi muscles, overlying fat and skin, are tunnelled under the skin below the axilla to create a new breast shape. This procedure can be used with or without an implant. Postoperative flap problems are rare, however patients sometimes experience a bulge under the axilla (Petit *et al.*, 2012).
- Transverse rectus abdominus myocutaneous flap (TRAM), which can be achieved with a free flap in which abdominal skin, fat, muscle and blood supply are detached and transposed to the breast area where the flap is reconnected to the blood supply at the axilla or sternum. This involves microsurgery and produces a better postoperative blood supply than a pedicled flap. Consequently, it has a longer procedure time of between six and eight hours.
- Pedicled TRAM flap involves taking the skin, fat and muscle from the abdomen, leaving the blood supply intact, tunnelled under the skin and formed into a new 'breast'. The operation time for this procedure is between four and five hours (Petit *et al.*, 2012).
- Further alternatives include DIEP flaps. In this case a flap of skin and fat, but not muscle, is transposed (Petit *et al.*, 2012). This procedure uses the deep inferior epigastric perforator blood vessels and has a procedure time of between six and eight hours. Finally, a SIEA flap involves the use of the superficial inferior epigastric artery flap.

Free TRAM, DIEP and SIEA flaps are microsurgery techniques and consequently involve long operation times. These are specialised surgery, undertaken in specialist centres, and are subject to long waiting lists. These procedures are not indicated for smokers or for patients with pre-existing co-morbidities such as diabetes, as their major risks are vascular insufficiency and consequent loss of the flap (Petit *et al.*, 2012). It must be borne in mind that a number of alternatives have been developed, often with the aim of benefiting certain patients such as those with larger breasts, or to reconstruct both breasts without implants. Some of these autogenous breast reconstruction techniques might have been suitable for Louise but because her children were young, to facilitate a quicker return to work and to minimise the amount of postoperative recovery time and scarring, she chose to have immediate reconstruction using tissue expanders, which were to be replaced by silicone prostheses during a second procedure.

3 **How would the perioperative team have prepared for Louise's care in the operating theatre?**

A A surgical brief was undertaken whereby the theatre team met, introduced themselves and identified the roles they would undertake that day. Each patient on the operating list was discussed, operative procedures clarified and any specific concerns or requirements relating to their perioperative care highlighted. This is in accordance with the Scottish Patient Safety Programme (SPSP), which aims to prevent adverse clinical incidents in healthcare. The SPSP encourages the formation of cohesive teams, information sharing and staff's 'ownership' of patient safety concerns, thereby ensuring that all team members act appropriately if they consider patient safety might be compromised.

Louise could reasonably be expected to be anxious and therefore the theatre atmosphere was quiet and calm to try to minimise extraneous factors that might compound her anxiety. The ambient theatre temperature was maintained at 22 degrees Celsius to avoid cooling the patient, thus minimising the risk of inadvertent hypothermia. The necessary instrumentation and tissue expanders were available, within date and in intact packaging, thus ensuring their sterility.

4 **Describe the most appropriate anaesthetic technique, and consider which drugs could be administered as part of the anaesthetic.**

A Louise was collected from the admissions unit where all appropriate preoperative checks were undertaken. She was transferred to the anaesthetic room, attached to monitoring, and her routine baseline recordings, ECG, SpO_2 and NIBP, were taken. A size 20G cannula was inserted into the dorsum of her left hand.

Louise was crying and expressed her anxiety, particularly about the anaesthetic and the possibility of awareness during the procedure. She was reassured that the risk of this was minimal and that she would be under constant close supervision to ascertain her physiological reaction to stimulus so that any signs of awareness would be identified and acted upon immediately.

Louise was pre-oxygenated and anaesthetised using:

- propofol 1%, which used as an induction agent has a rapid distribution and therefore wears off quickly at the end of the procedure
- fentanyl, which is an analgesic that obtunds the laryngeal reflexes, thereby minimising the risk of laryngospasm on induction, and

- vecuronium, which allowed Louise to be intubated and ventilated; vecuronium is a non-depolarising muscle relaxant that does not normally cause histamine release or adverse cardiac effects (Hunter, 2007); it can be reversed immediately using sugammadex (Caldwell and Miller, 2009).

She was intubated with a size 7 mm cuffed endotracheal tube and was commenced on intermittent positive pressure ventilation. Her end tidal carbon dioxide was continually monitored to ensure that her airway remained patent and gaseous exchange was taking place. Anaesthesia was maintained using sevoflurane, which is useful as it has a rapid uptake and a relatively quick reversal. Furthermore, it is also non-irritant, which further minimises the risk of laryngospasm.

Morphine 10 mg and fentanyl 100 micrograms were administered as intraoperative analgesia. A patient-controlled analgesia device (PCA) with morphine 50 mg in 100 ml saline was prescribed and prepared for postoperative pain control. This would enable Louise to self-administer her postoperative analgesia, thereby empowering her to actively participate in her care.

Louise's temperature was monitored using an oesophageal probe. This provides a continuous temperature recording and was selected because of the extensive nature of surgery, whereby the large wound exposure might give rise to a significant drop in core temperature. This would predispose Louise to a range of complications, such as wound infection, postoperative bleeding, decreased drug metabolism and prolonged recovery time (Hooper *et al.*, 2009).

5   **Describe how Louise was prepared for surgery, paying particular attention to patient positioning and risk assessment.**

A   Louise was positioned supine with her arms on arm boards, at a less than 90-degree angle to avoid damage to the brachial plexus. The risks of pressure sores associated with supine positioning were minimised by the use of pillows, gel pad mattress, heel pads and arm board pads. Scottish Intercollegiate Guidelines Network (SIGN) Guideline 122 states that patients admitted to hospital for major surgery should have their risk of venous thromboembolism (VTE) assessed and be treated accordingly. Patients who are having surgery are at an increased risk of developing VTE due to pooling of blood in the deep veins, especially of the calves, because of inactivity during and immediately following surgery. Static blood has an increased propensity for clot formation, particularly around the valves in the deep veins.

This risk of development of VTE was addressed by the application of intermittent pneumatic compression leggings, which continuously inflate and deflate thereby compressing the muscles of the calf, stimulating the return of venous blood to the heart, preventing venous stasis and minimising the risk of formation of deep vein thrombosis. In addition, Louise was fitted with graduated elastic compression stockings, which she would wear until she was fully mobile postoperatively.

Louise's temperature control was addressed in various ways. Intravenous fluids were warmed and a lower body forced air warming blanket was applied. These measures combined ensured that her core body temperature was maintained within normal limits.

A prophylactic antibiotic, Augmentin®, was prescribed and administered intravenously within 30 minutes of skin incision, to minimise the risk of postoperative surgical site infection in line with SIGN Guideline 104, *Antibiotic Prophylaxis in Surgery* (Scottish Intercollegiate Guidelines Network, 2008). The development of surgical site infection might lead to the subsequent need for removal of the tissue expanders.

Stop and think

How would Louise's age and choice of reconstructive options impact upon the surgical intervention at this stage?

Bilateral skin-sparing prophylactic mastectomies were performed to accommodate the insertion of tissue expanders. The tissue expanders were placed under the pectoral muscles and the inflation ports were placed under the skin of the chest. These procedures necessitated the use of plastic surgery instrumentation in order to optimise the postoperative cosmetic outcome. The tissue expanders' reference and lot numbers were recorded in the patient's notes and operation register so the implants could be identified should any subsequent patient safety issues arise.

---

6 **What type of wound closure, dressing and drainage would be most appropriate?**

A A low-vacuum suction drain was inserted into each wound site to drain any bleeding or seroma, to minimise the risk of postoperative wound infection. The wound was closed with continuous absorbable monofilament suture to minimise scarring and negate the need for postoperative suture removal. Transparent adhesive dressings with integrated absorbent pads were applied so that the wound could be observed for signs of bleeding, seroma or infection. The dressings were water repellent, allowing Louise to bathe postoperatively without disturbing the wound sites.

7 **What would be your priorities for caring for Louise in the post-anaesthetic care unit?**

A Louise was extubated and transferred to the PACU. She was attached to electrocardiograph, non-invasive blood pressure and oxygen saturation monitoring. Louise was assessed and observed using the ABCDE approach to patient assessment. Oxygen was administered at 5 litres per minute via a face mask. Her airway was self-maintained and her physiological observations were within normal limits. Her temperature was recorded at regular intervals to ensure that normothermia was maintained.

She was placed in the semi-recumbent position to try to minimise postoperative pain from pressure on the wound sites. Her pain was assessed using a numerical rating scale, which is useful for assessing pain and evaluating the efficacy of pain-relieving strategies, particularly in situations where the patient either will not or cannot tolerate lengthy questioning (Brown, 2008). Once her pain rating was within acceptable limits, Louise had her PCA device attached and, by activating it as required, she maintained her pain score within tolerable limits. The PCA allowed Louise to control the administration of pain relief to manage her own pain. This was useful as there is no reliable way of predicting what the patient's need for postoperative analgesia is likely to be. Therefore, enabling Louise to control her postoperative pain gave her the opportunity to manage it according to her individual needs. The use of PCA devices is also thought to enhance the placebo effect that comes from the autonomy it brings (Power and Atcheson, 2007). PCA devices are not recommended for everybody, however, as the patient's cognitive ability must be such that they understand how and when to use the device for it to provide a satisfactory level of pain control (Power and Atcheson, 2007). Louise reported this method of pain control added to her self-determination, which let her be an active participant in, rather than a passive recipient of, her care.

Louise suffered postoperative nausea and vomited. Her privacy was ensured using screens. She was offered oral toilet following emesis. Her anaesthetic and prescription chart were checked to determine which anti-emetics had been administered and prescribed. Louise had not had any anti-emetics administered in theatre. Ondansetron 4 mg was prescribed and administered intravenously to control nausea and vomiting, with the desired effect. Her wounds were observed for signs of bleeding, discolouration or swelling, which might indicate the presence of seroma. Her drains were clamped off for 30 minutes postoperatively to produce a tamponade effect in her wounds. After 30 minutes, the drains were opened and their return, which was minimal, was observed and documented.

Louise was provided with a calm, therapeutic environment in the immediate postoperative period to facilitate recovery from surgery and anaesthesia. She continued to cry despite reporting her pain as not significant, but did admit to feeling very emotional. She was provided with psychological support by encouraging her to talk about her concerns. She discussed her worry about her children's long-term prognoses and talked about her sister's death. When Louise was fully recovered, with all her physiological parameters within normal limits, she was discharged from PACU to a general surgical ward.

8   **Consider the ongoing care that Louise will require to achieve a satisfactory patient outcome.**

A   Louise remained in hospital for several days and had analgesia to facilitate early mobility. Her wounds were dry and her drains removed on her third postoperative day when drainage was less than 35 ml per day. She was then discharged home. Her sutures were removed seven days post-surgery. Subsequently, Louise had saline injected at regular one- to two-week intervals to create space for the anatomical silicone implants. Her return for surgery enabled the correction of any aesthetic issues and thereby improvement of the appearance of the reconstructed breasts.

Following her second surgery, Louise is very satisfied with the appearance of her reconstructions and is reassured that her subsequent risk of developing breast cancer is significantly reduced (Nestle-Kramling and Kühn, 2012). Unfortunately Louise continues to experience left-sided pain and altered sensation, which she self-manages with analgesics and does not consider to be life limiting. Power and Atcheson (2007), however, advise that although acute postoperative pain usually resolves relatively quickly, there is a significant incidence of chronic pain following some surgical procedures, including mastectomy. Louise has not been referred to a chronic pain specialist but may benefit from this if her symptoms persist or become problematic.

In addition, a pain management programme provided by a specialist multidisciplinary team can provide information and education about pain and its management.

q **Reflect upon the patient journey and the difficult decisions that Louise has had to make in the context of her BRCA2 gene mutation.**

A Louise chose prophylactic surgery, believing that the benefits of minimising her subsequent risk of breast cancer outweighed any risks of surgery. She was determined to survive to raise her children. Body image concerns were dwarfed by her resolve to maximise her chance of survival, hence her decision not to have nipple-sparing surgery.

Louise's main concern for the future is whether to have her children tested for the BRCA gene mutation. Throughout her decision making and subsequent surgical procedures, she has explained her experiences to her children in simple terms. She believes that, by doing so, she has given her children a positive role model and a constructive experience of prophylactic surgery.

She has also decided to undergo prophylactic bilateral salpingo-oophorectomies to minimise her subsequent risk of contracting ovarian cancer. Kurian and Ford (2011) recommend risk-reducing bilateral salpingo-oophorectomy for all BRCA1- and BRCA2-positive women by or before the age of 40 because of their high risk of ovarian cancer and the lack of effective screening alternatives. Louise will wait until she is 35 and then undergo this further prophylactic procedure.

REFERENCES AND FURTHER READING

Benedet, R.D. (2011) The role of the specialist breast nurse, in Dirbas, F.M. and Scott-Conner, C.E.H. (eds) *Breast Surgical Techniques and Interdisciplinary Management*. New York: Springer Science + Business Media.

Brown, D.N. (2008) Pain assessment in the recovery room. *Journal of Perioperative Practice*, **18**(11): 480–489.

Caldwell, J.E. and Miller, R.D. (2009) Clinical implications of sugammadex. *Anaesthesia*, **64**: 66–72. Available online at: http://onlinelibrary.wiley.com/doi/10.1111/j.1365–2044.2008. 05872.x/ full (accessed 1 September 2015).

Cancer Research UK (2012a) Breast reconstruction using body tissue. Available online at: www.cancerresearchuk.org/about-cancer/type/breast-cancer/treatment/surgery/ reconstruction/breast-reconstruction-using-body-tissue (accessed 31 August 2014).

Cancer Research UK (2012b) Breast reconstruction using implants. Available online at: www. cancerresearchuk.org/about-cancer/type/breast-cancer/treatment/surgery/reconstruction/ breast-reconstruction-using-implants (accessed 31 August 2014).

DellaCroce, F.J. and Wolfe, E.T. (2013) Breast reconstruction. *Surgical Clinics of North America*, **93**(2): 445–454.

Hooper, V.D., Chard, R., Clifford, T., Fetzer, S., Fossum, S., Godden, B., Martinez, E.A., Noble, K.A., O'Brien, D., Odom-Forren, J., Perterson, C. and Ross, J. (2009) ASPAN's evidence-based clinical practice guideline for the promotion of perioperative normothermia. *Journal of Perianaesthesia Nursing*, **24**(5): 271–287. Available online at: www.jopan.org/article/ S1089–9472(09)00339–6/fulltext (accessed 31 August 2015).

Hoskins, L.M. and Greene, M.H. (2012) Anticipatory loss and early mastectomy for young female BRCA1 or 2 mutation carriers. *Qualitative Health Research*, **22**(12): 1633–1646.

Hunter, J.M. (2007) Muscle function and neuromuscular blockade, in Aitkenhead, A.R., Smith, G. and Rowbotham, D.J. (eds) *Textbook of Anaesthesia* (5th edn). Edinburgh: Churchill Livingstone.

Kurian, A.W. and Ford, J.M. (2011) Identification and management of women at high familial risk for breast cancer, in Dirbas, F.M. and Scott-Conner, C.E.H. (eds) *Breast Surgical Techniques and Interdisciplinary Management*. New York: Springer Science + Business Media.

Macmillan Cancer Support (2014) Breast reconstruction using an implant. Available online at: www.macmillan.org.uk/information-and-support/treating/surgery/types-of-breast-reconstruction/Breast-reconstruction-using-an-implant.html (accessed 31 August 2015).

Medicines and Healthcare Products Regulatory Agency (2012) Breast implants: information for women considering breast implants. Available online at: www.wales.nhs.uk/sites3/Documents/456/MHRA%20Breast%20Implants%20-%20information%20for%20women%20considering%20breast%20implants1.pdf (accessed 25 January 2016).

Nestle-Kramling, C. and Kühn, T. (2012) Role of breast surgery in BRCA mutation carriers. *Breast Care*, **7**(5): 378–382.

Niemeyer, M., Paepke, S., Schmid, R., Plattner, B., Müller, D. and Kiechle, M. (2011) Extended indications for nipple-sparing mastectomy. *The Breast Journal*, **17**(3). Available online at: http://onlinelibrary.wiley.com/doi/10.1111/j.1524–4741.2011.01079.x/pdf (accessed 31 August 2015).

Petit, J.-Y., Rietjens, M., Lohsiriwat, V., Rey, P., Garusi, C., De Lorenzi, F., Martella, S., Manconi, A., Barbieri, B. and Clough, K.B. (2012) Update on breast reconstruction techniques and indications. *World Journal of Surgery*. Available online at: http://link.springer.com/article/10.1007%2Fs00268–012–1486–3/fulltext.html (accessed 17 April 2014).

Power, I. and Atcheson, R. (2007) Postoperative pain, in Aitkenhead, A.R., Smith, G. and Rowbotham, D.J. (eds) *Textbook of Anaesthesia* (5th edn). Edinburgh: Churchill Livingstone.

Samson, A., DiMillo, J., Thériault, A., Lowry, S., Corsini, L., Verma, S. and Tomiak, E. (2014) Living with the BRCA1 and BRCA2 genetic mutation: learning how to adapt to a virtual chronic illness. *Psychology, Health & Medicine*, **19**(1): 103–114.

Scottish Intercollegiate Guidelines Network (SIGN) (2008) *Guideline 104: Antibiotic Prophylaxis in Surgery*. Edinburgh: SIGN. Available online at: www.sign.ac.uk/pdf/sign104.pdf (accessed 9 March 2014).

Scottish Intercollegiate Guidelines Network (SIGN) (2010) *Guideline 122: Prevention and Management of Venous Thromboembolism*. Edinburgh: SIGN. Available online at: www.sign.ac.uk/guidelines/fulltext/122/index.html (accessed 14 April 2014).

Scottish Patient Safety Programme (n.d.) Available online at: www.scottishpatientsafetyprogramme.scot.nhs.uk/programme (accessed 2 March 2014).

Smith, E.C. (2012) An overview of hereditary breast and ovarian cancer syndrome. *Journal of Midwifery & Women's Health*, **57**(6): 577–584.

Sweetland, H.M. (2006) Breast reconstruction. *Women's Health Medicine*, **3**(1): 34–35.

Caesarean section: the care of Mary-Jane James

Hannah Abbott

INTRODUCTION AND LEARNING OUTCOMES

Caesarean section (C-section) is the surgical delivery of a neonate and is becoming increasingly common, accounting for 26.2% of deliveries in NHS hospitals in 2013–14 (Health and Social Care Information Centre, 2015). There are a number of indications for C-section and these will generally inform the urgency of the surgery: from life-saving C-sections required urgently, to elective surgery by maternal request. While operating departments perform C-sections on a regular basis, it is important to remember that this is abdominal surgery that presents a number of unique risks and hence the perioperative team need to ensure that each patient is assessed prior to and throughout their perioperative journey.

By the end of case study you will be able to:

- explain the physiological changes related to pregnancy and the impact upon perioperative care
- discuss the evidence-based interventions required for the care of the patient undergoing C-section
- discuss the complexities of involving a birthing partner in the care of the patient.

Case outline

Mary-Jane James is a 34-year-old female who lives with her husband Salvatore in a large town within commuting distance of London, where she works as a corporate lawyer; her husband is in finance and also works in the City. Mary-Jane has been married for four years and is 39 weeks pregnant with their second child after their first child was stillborn 18 months previously following a vaginal delivery. This is identified by the Teardrop sticker on Mary-Jane's notes; these stickers were designed to alert staff that the patient had a baby that died, so that they are aware and can be sensitive to this when conversing with the patient (Sands, 2014).

Mary-Jane also had an unplanned pregnancy when she was 19, during her first year at university, and had suction termination of pregnancy (STOP) under general anaesthetic (GA) at 10 weeks' gestation. Mary-Jane felt that, as a student, she was not able to cope with a child and feared reprisal from her family, who would have disapproved of a pregnancy outside of marriage; consequently her termination was performed under clause C (Section 1 (1) of the 1967 Abortion Act) as it was considered that continuing with the pregnancy would involve greater risk to Mary-Jane's physical or mental health than a termination; the majority (98% in 2014) of terminations in the UK are performed under clause C (DH, 2015). Salvatore however is not aware that Mary-Jane has had a termination previously, as he is a practising Roman Catholic who does not believe in the termination of pregnancy, and Mary-Jane fears that he would disapprove of her actions and also of the fact that she had not told him earlier in their ten-year relationship. All staff caring for Mary-Jane must therefore uphold their legal and professional duty to maintain patient confidentiality, and must therefore be aware that, while it is important to involve Salvatore, they don't assume that Mary-Jane is willing to have her care and past medical history discussed while he is present.

Mary-Jane and her husband started trying to conceive three months following the stillbirth of their first child, after having discussed this with their obstetrician, as they felt that they were ready to have another child. Following her first missed period, Mary-Jane took a home pregnancy test, which was positive, and made an appointment to see her general practitioner (GP) to initiate her antenatal care; she also received initial health advice relating to folic acid supplements, lifestyle factors during pregnancy (for example, smoking and alcohol consumption), antenatal screening and food hygiene (NICE, 2008). Mary-Jane was booked for antenatal appointments approximately every month; these included routine tests and discussion relating to pregnancy and birth – for example, the foetal development, nutrition and diet, delivery, care of the neonate, breastfeeding and post-partum care (NICE, 2008). As part of routine antenatal screening Mary-Jane had a 'combined test' for Down's syndrome at 12 weeks. This consists of a scan to test nuchal translucency, and a blood test to test levels of beta-human chorionic gonadotrophin and pregnancy-associated plasma protein-A (NICE, 2008). Mary-Jane's results were low risk, so no further testing for Down's syndrome was required. She also had two ultrasound scans as part of her routine antenatal care, the first at 12 weeks, which determined gestational age, and a further, more detailed, scan at 20 weeks where they were also able to determine the gender. In addition to these routine scans, Mary-Jane and Salvatore also opted to have a private 4D scan, which allowed detailed visualisation of the baby, including facial features.

Mary-Jane specifically requested a C-section as, following her previous stillbirth, she felt that another labour would prove too stressful and would trigger memories of her recent bereavement. In accordance with NICE (2011) guidelines, Mary-Jane's reasons for requesting C-section were explored, along with an explanation of the risks and benefits. Following these discussions C-section remained the preferred option and therefore an elective C-section was scheduled at a mutually agreed time.

> **Stop and think**
>
> What would your initial plan of care be for Mary-Jane? You should consider her physiological care needs, while also considering her psychosocial care. Also try to consider how you will involve Salvatore while ensuring Mary-Jane's confidentiality is protected.

1 **What physiological changes occur in pregnancy? You should focus on the changes that affect the respiratory and gastrointestinal systems, and consider how these would impact upon perioperative care.**

A There are a number of changes to the airway during pregnancy, which increase the risk of difficult intubation. The upper airway is oedematous, which is increased in pre-eclampsia or in women who have been actively pushing, and the tongue and epiglottis are enlarged. This adversely impacts visualisation of the larynx during laryngoscopy; this is compounded by increased breast size, which may obstruct the position of the laryngoscope. The pregnant patient will also desaturate faster, as their functional residual capacity is reduced and their metabolic rate (and hence oxygen demand) is increased (Drake and Drake, 2009).

In addition to changes to the airway, there are also changes to the gastrointestinal system, which necessitate a rapid-sequence induction for all patients undergoing a C-section under general anaesthesia, irrespective of fasting status. Increased progesterone in early pregnancy causes relaxation of smooth muscle, including the lower oesophageal sphincter and, when combined with the abdominal mass of the gravid uterus, this increases the risk of regurgitation and aspiration; in addition, gastric contents have a lower pH (AnaesthesiaUK, 2006). Patients who are actively labouring will also have delayed gastric emptying; this is due to a combination of anxiety, pain and resulting opioid administration.

The relaxation of muscle tone in pregnancy due to increased progesterone also impacts blood pressure as the blood vessels dilate and hence normal blood pressure is reduced; this is most noticeable in the second trimester, and Mary-Jane found that she often felt faint and dizzy when she was 15–18 weeks pregnant; this is counteracted in the third trimester by the increased plasma volume, which restores blood pressure to the patient's normal (pre-pregnancy level) (Passmore, 2014).

2 **How would Mary-Jane be prepared preoperatively?**

A Mary-Jane was admitted on to the obstetric ward on the morning of her surgery, which is usual for elective C-section. She was advised to shower on the morning of her surgery, but was explicitly advised not to shave her bikini line, as shaving prior to surgery has been associated with an increased risk of infection. Mary-Jane was required to be nil by mouth for a minimum of six hours for solids and milk, and two hours for water and clear fluids (RCN, 2005), and so had not eaten since going to bed but was able to have a drink first thing in the morning. At the time of admission, routine baseline observations were performed including heart rate, blood pressure and oxygen saturations; these were all within normal limits, although Mary-Jane's heart rate and blood pressure were slightly higher than her normal, which was attributed to anxiety. Mary-Jane had a preoperative haemoglobin assessment, which showed that she was not anaemic and, as she has been fit and well throughout her pregnancy, she did not require any further preoperative blood tests (NICE, 2011). Specific to C-section admissions, abdominal palpation is undertaken to confirm the foetal presentation, which in this case was cephalic presentation, and the foetal heart rate is auscultated. Mary-Jane was also measured for and fitted with graduated compression stockings as pregnancy increases the risk of deep venous thromboembolism and hence Mary-Jane will be advised to wear these throughout her stay in hospital and to mobilise as soon as possible.

3   **How would you prepare the theatre environment for this case? What specific equipment is required in the theatre for C-section?**

A   Mary-Jane will undergo surgery in the designated obstetric theatre, which is fully prepared for C-section and instrumental delivery procedures. The operating table in the obstetric theatre must be able to support a minimum of 160 kg and therefore theatre practitioners must be aware of the maximum weight limit for the specific table and where an alternative can be found for patients exceeding this (AAGBI, 2005). The theatre must also be equipped for adverse obstetric incidents – this includes having a rapid infuser to transfuse high volumes of warmed blood and fluids – and a difficult intubation trolley, where a full range of airway adjuncts including endotracheal tubes and laryngeal masks must be available (AAGBI, 2005); this trolley is usually checked on a daily basis and typically has a copy of the local failed obstetric intubation drill attached to it. The theatre must also have monitoring equipment available, including ECG, NIBP, pulse oximetry, capnography, anaesthetic gas analyser, disconnection monitor, airway pressure monitor, invasive monitoring and nerve stimulator (to monitor neuromuscular blockade); in addition there must be temperature monitoring equipment and a forced air warmer with appropriate blankets (AAGBI, 2005).

This theatre will also have the appropriate equipment to care for the neonate; this will typically be contained as part of the Resuscitaire. The Resuscitaire has piped and cylinder oxygen, and pipeline suction, which must be checked daily, in addition to checking that the light and heating platform is functional. The responsibility for performing these checks varies between hospitals, however it is essential that they are performed. The Resuscitaire is also stocked with neonatal resuscitation equipment including a bag-valve mask, a range of endotracheal tubes, laryngoscopes, suction catheters, cannulas and neonatal resuscitation drug box; in addition, naloxone is normally stored in the Resuscitaire to treat neonatal bradypnea or apnoea due to maternal opioids. Prior to Mary-Jane's C-section, the Resuscitaire had been checked by the duty midwife, towels had been placed on the cot section and the heating platform had been turned on ready to receive the baby immediately after delivery.

4   **What anaesthetic do you think would be most appropriate for Mary-Jane and why? You should consider the evidence base in addition to holistic care considerations.**

A   An anaesthetic assessment was conducted by the anaesthetist as discussed in the Introduction to this book; however, it was important that discussion regarding previous anaesthesia was handled sensitively as, while it was essential to gain this informa-tion, it was imperative that Mary-Jane's confidentiality was protected. As part of this assessment the anaesthetic options were discussed and it was agreed that Mary-Jane would have a spinal anaesthetic, which is considered the anaesthetic technique of choice for C-section, as NICE (2011) reports that this is associated with reduced maternal and neonatal morbidity compared with general anaesthesia. This is not sup-ported by the most recent Cochrane Review, however, which concluded that there was insufficient evidence for the superiority of either technique with regard to mor-tality (neonatal or maternal) and hence considered that other outcomes would influ-ence the most appropriate technique – for example, maternal blood loss, which is reduced with spinal anaesthesia (Afolobi, Lesi and Merah, 2012). Despite this, however, spinal is associated with less maternal risk, predominantly related to the establish-ment of an airway, as the incidence of difficult intubation is considerably higher in pregnant women, and therefore the administration of a spinal anaesthetic virtually eliminates the risk of aspiration and allows the patient to maintain their own airway. There are also a number of holistic benefits to spinal anaesthesia for Mary-Jane, as both she and Salvatore are able to 'experience' the delivery and hold the baby soon after delivery, there is less postoperative 'hangover' and spinal also offers postop-erative analgesia.

The spinal anaesthesia was administered in theatre, with Mary-Jane sitting on the operating table, as this facilitates positioning quickly after spinal administration. Mary-Jane is asked to 'curl her back outwards' as this slightly increases the space between vertebrae, allowing access – although Mary-Jane found establishing and maintaining this position difficult as 'the bump was in the way'. The skin was prepared using chlorhexidine and a fenestrated spinal drape was applied to her back, thus creating a sterile field. A 25 gauge Whitacre spinal needle was used for the spinal as this has a 'pencil point', which is non-cutting and atraumatic; this is to reduce the incidence of dural headache because the needle separates the fibres of the dura and hence, when the needle is withdrawn, the fibres should be self-sealing thus prevent-ing leakage of cerebrospinal fluid (CSF). The intrathecal analgesic combination for Mary-Jane was 2.5 ml of 0.5% hyperbaric ('heavy') bupivacaine with 300 mcg diamor-phine (Eldridge, 2011). Hyperbaric bupivacaine is a long-acting local anaesthetic agent that has glucose added to it, thus reducing the risk of a high spinal, which could compromise respiration. Diamorphine was added to the spinal dose as this can increase the quality of the analgesia in addition to providing postoperative analgesia; the main advantage of diamorphine is a high lipid solubility, which allows it to cross the blood–brain barrier rapidly and means that smaller doses can be administered (in comparison to morphine) (Rang *et al.*, 2011).

5   **Why would Mary-Jane be administered intravenous fluids as part of her perioperative care?**

A   Throughout her care in the operating department Mary-Jane was administered crystalloid fluids via a 16G cannula. This is to alleviate some of the hypotension result-ing from the vascular dilatation due to the spinal; this hypotension most commonly causes nausea and vomiting. The administration of IV fluids alone, however, has been shown to be insufficient to eliminate spinal-induced maternal hypotension and therefore the anaesthetist was prepared to treat any presenting hypotension with ephedrine or phenylephrine (Cyna et al., 2006).

6 **How was Mary-Jane positioned for her surgery and why?**

A Mary-Jane was positioned supine on the operating table with a 15-degree left lateral tilt; this is to alleviate pressure from the gravid uterus upon the inferior vena cava, as this can cause hypotension. Salvatore is seated next to Mary-Jane facing her head and away from the incision, this allows him to be present for the delivery but minimises his view of the surgical procedure. A screen is also fixed to the table; this serves a dual purpose, both to keep the surgical drapes away from Mary-Jane's face and also to prevent her seeing any of the surgery. Some surgeons and anaesthetists offer the patient the option to lower the screen at the point of delivery so that they can watch, however Mary-Jane declined this option as she 'is not good with the sight of blood' and did not feel comfortable with this option.

7 **How was Mary-Jane prepared for surgery?**

A Mary-Jane was catheterised using a Foley catheter to prevent over-distension of the bladder attributed to regional anaesthesia (NICE, 2011) and this will remain in situ until Mary-Jane has regained all motor function and is able to mobilise sufficiently to safely walk to the toilet. Once the skin preparation and draping were complete the anaesthetist gave permission for the surgery to commence, and informed Mary-Jane and Salvatore that they were starting the procedure; Mary-Jane was made aware that, while she should not feel any sharp pain, she may still feel some movement and pressure; this is important so that the patient is appropriately prepared.

8 **What surgical instruments are prepared specific to the C-section procedure?**

A The surgical team prepared the surgical instruments ensuring the use of aseptic technique throughout. There is a designated C-section set, which will be used for all C-sections and, while there may be some local variations, all will contain generic instruments for abdominal surgery, including blade handles, dissecting scissors, artery forceps, toothed and non-toothed forceps, and needle holders. In addition, there are some instruments that are unique to C-section; these are commonly the Doyen's (or other large curved) retractor, which is used to expose the bladder and lower segment by placing it under the symphysis pubis, and Green-Armytage forceps, which are applied to the edges of the uterine incision after delivery, and used to control blood loss and for alignment prior to uterine closure (Shields and Werder, 2002). Obstetric forceps are also typically found on C-section trays, however these should not be used routinely as their effect on neonatal mortality is unknown; they will be used only if the delivery of the head proves to be difficult (NICE, 2011); consequently, they may be required urgently and must therefore be dissembled ready for application to the head if required. In addition to the surgical instrumentation, the surgical team must ensure that there is a suitably large plastic bowl for the placenta, as the midwifery team will wish to examine this post-surgery to ensure it is intact. It is also important that there are sufficient cord clamps – two clamps will be required for each baby – however in the event of multiple deliveries the number of cord clamps is usually used to denote the order of delivery – for example, 'Baby one' with one cord clamp and 'Baby two' with two cord clamps.

q **What does the surgical procedure involve?**

A The usual approach for C-section is a transverse abdominal incision as this results in improved cosmetic results and reduced postoperative pain compared with a midline incision; in accordance with NICE (2011) guidelines, a Joel-Cohen incision is used for Mary-Jane's surgery, this is 'a straight skin incision, 3 cm above the symphysis pubis'; 'subsequent layers are opened bluntly and, if necessary, extended with scissors and not a knife' (NICE, 2011: 21). The other commonly used transverse incision for C-section is the Pfannenstiel incision, however the Joel-Cohen incision has been shown to be superior for reduced febrile morbidity, reduced postoperative analgesia, reduced blood loss (estimated), and also reduced times for surgery, delivery and postoperative length of stay (Abalos, 2009).

When the team are preparing to incise the uterus they warn Mary-Jane that she will hear the suction shortly as 'her waters break' and the amniotic fluid is released, and also that she will feel pressure as the surgical assistant applies downward pressure to assist in the delivery. The surgeon delivered the baby head first and the time of delivery was recorded; the cord was clamped with a disposable cord clamp (approximately 2 cm from the base of the umbilical cord) and Kocher's forceps were used as the second clamp – the umbilical cord was then cut between the two clamps (Shields and Werder, 2002). The surgeon lifted the baby above the drape to show Mary-Jane and Salvatore that they have a son; the baby was then passed to the midwife to undertake an initial examination of the baby at the Resuscitaire. Following the safe delivery of the baby, the placenta was delivered by controlled traction on the umbilical cord and 5 IU of intravenous oxytocin was administered; this decreases blood loss by stimulating uterine contraction (NICE, 2011).

10 **Discuss the closure of the cavities and the evidence base that underpins this.**

A The uterus was closed with a double layer of sutures; this was performed with the uterus within the peritoneum as NICE (2011) does not advise exteriorisation of the uterus as this does not offer improved postoperative outcomes and may result in increased postoperative pain. There are no peritoneal sutures as these have not been shown to improve patient outcomes and, as Mary-Jane has less than 2 cm subcutaneous fat, there is no requirement to suture the subcutaneous tissue (NICE, 2011). The skin was closed with a subcutaneous non-absorbable suture as sutures have been suggested as preferable to skin staples following C-section, as staples have been associated with a higher incidence of wound infection or separation (NICE, 2013). A permeable self-adhesive dressing is applied to the abdominal wound and a sanitary towel placed over the perineal area prior to transferring Mary-Jane back to her bed.

11 **What are the requirements for the standard of care provided in the PACU following C-section?**

A The whole family was transferred into the designated obstetric PACU area; at this hospital this is a private room adjacent to the main PACU, however this will vary between hospitals. Although Mary-Jane had regional anaesthesia, it must be remembered that she has still undergone abdominal surgery and should have the same standard of care as any other perioperative patient, including during her time in the PACU. As such, a designated PACU practitioner provides her post-anaesthetic care, as midwives are not generally qualified for PACU care of obstetric patients unless they have undertaken additional PACU education and training (AAGBI, 2005).

12   **What specific assessments are required in the PACU following C-section?**

A   Mary-Jane has the normal PACU assessment and monitoring, as detailed in the Introduction, which shows observations within the normal range. As the spinal anaesthetic had contained diamorphine, it was necessary to monitor respiratory rate and sedation score for 12 hours postoperatively as opioids have a depressive effect on the respiratory system. Mary-Jane's pain was monitored using the numerical rating scale and she rated her pain as a 2. This can be attributed to the residual spinal blockade and the administration of per rectum diclofenac at the end of surgery. Mary-Jane is advised that she should report any increases in her pain level and shouldn't wait for pain to become severe before requesting analgesics; pain assessment will be ongoing for a minimum of 12 hours postoperatively. The recovery practitioner checked Mary-Jane's abdominal wound as is normal practice for all patients in the PACU, however following C-section it is also important to check for excessive per vagina (PV) blood loss.

13   **How can Mary-Jane be supported to bond with her baby in the PACU?**

A   The period in the PACU is an important time for Mary-Jane to bond with her baby and, as part of this, skin-to-skin contact is encouraged. It is usual to allow the mother the opportunity to breastfeed in this period if they wish to, especially as it has been recognised that mothers who have a C-section delivery may initiate breastfeeding later than those who have a vaginal delivery. Mary-Jane declines this, however, as she has decided that she does not wish to breastfeed and has brought bottles and formula with her, and will commence feeding when she returns to the ward. It is important therefore that the PACU practitioner is sensitive to the patient's needs, and does not inadvertently make the patient feel that breastfeeding is required or expected. Mary-Jane and Salvatore however want to use some of this time to take some photographs and to have their baby weighed and measured as this is facilitated within this PACU.

14   **What continued care does Mary-Jane require when she returns to the ward?**

A   On her return to the ward, Mary-Jane was monitored in accordance with NICE (2011) guidelines, which require observations every 30 minutes for the first two hours and then, as Mary-Jane's observations were stable, on an hourly basis. Mary-Jane and Salvatore also spent some time with their baby who was dressed in the outfit they had chosen. Mary-Jane was encouraged to eat and drink normally as she wanted, although she was advised to ensure she had sufficient fibre to prevent constipation. Mary-Jane was in hospital for three days, which is usual following C-section with 56.3% of patients staying three or more days following surgery and 21.2% staying five or more days (Health and Social Care Information Centre, 2013).

15 **What care advice must Mary-Jane receive before she is discharged from hospital?**

A Mary-Jane was advised that she can return to normal activities as she feels able, although she must be careful to avoid lifting heavy loads and must ensure she checks her insurance policy before driving again. Mary-Jane was also offered contraceptive advice before leaving hospital and was advised that, as she does not want another pregnancy, she must use contraception from 21 days post-delivery. She subsequently decides to have an intra-uterine system (IUS), which can be fitted from 28 days after C-section (FPA, 2014). A follow-up appointment is booked for six to eight weeks postoperatively and, following this, Mary-Jane intends to return to work.

16 **Reflect upon this case study and consider how you as an ODP can make a positive contribution to improving Mary-Jane's and Salvatore's experience within the perioperative environment. You should also consider any challenges and how they may be overcome.**

A While Mary-Jane was the patient, and hence her care was the priority, it was also important for the team to support Salvatore, as attending theatre with a partner can be a daunting experience. The team were careful to ensure that they informed Salvatore of where to position himself and to alert them should he feel unwell. Once the examination of the newborn was completed the midwife brought him to Salvatore to hold; skin-to-skin contact with the mother is also encouraged at this time, although it is not always feasible.

The theatre team offered to take a photograph of the new family as soon as possible after delivery, as parents often bring a camera to theatre. The theatre team should also be sensitive to any specific requests relating to the delivery and try to accommodate these where possible – for example, some parents will bring music they would like to play, while others may want silence during the delivery. C-section therefore presents the challenge of delivering a personalised, intimate experience for the parents, but within the confines of a clinical setting; consequently it is essential that practitioners deliver an individualised plan of perioperative care for each patient.

REFERENCES AND FURTHER READING

Abalos, E. (2009) Surgical techniques for Caesarean section: RHL commentary. *The WHO Reproductive Health Library*. Geneva: World Health Organization.

Afolobi, B.B., Lesi, A.F.E. and Merah, N.A. (2012) Regional versus general anaesthesia for caesarean section. Review. The Cochrane Library.

AnaesthesiaUK (2006) Physiological changes of pregnancy. Available online at: www.frca.co.uk/article.aspx?articleid=100601 (accessed 18 September 2014).

Association of Anaesthetists of Great Britain and Ireland (AAGBI) (2005) *OAA/AAGBI Guidelines for Obstetric Anaesthetic Services* (rev. edn). London: AAGBI.

Cyna, A.M., Andrew, M., Emmett, R.S., Middleton, P. and Simmons, S.W. (2006) Techniques for preventing hypotension during spinal anaesthesia for caesarean section. Review. The Cochrane Library.

Department of Health (DH) (2015) Abortion statistics, England and Wales: 2014. Available online at: www.gov.uk (accessed 27 October 2015).

Drake, M. and Drake, E. (2009) Obstetric anaesthesia: recent advances and ongoing issues. *Technic: The Journal of Operating Department Practice*, **1**(1): 8–9.

Eldridge, J. (2011) Obstetric anaesthesia and analgesia, in Allman, K.G. and Wilson, I.H. (eds) *Oxford Handbook of Anaesthesia* (3rd edn). Oxford: Oxford University Press.

FPA (2014) Your guide to contraceptive choices – after you've had your baby. Available online at: www.fpa.org.uk (accessed 27 October 2015).

Health and Social Care Information Centre (2013) Hospital episode statistics, NHS maternity statistics 2012–13. Available online at: www.hscic.gov.uk/catalogue/PUB12744/nhs-mate-eng-2012–13-summ-repo-rep.pdf (accessed 14 September 2014).

Health and Social Care Information Centre (2015) Hospital episode statistics, NHS maternity statistics – England, 2013–14. Available online at: www.hscic.gov.uk (accessed 27 October 2015).

National Institute for Health and Clinical Excellence (NICE) (2008) Antenatal care. *NICE Clinical Guideline 62* (last modified June 2010). Available online at: www.nice.org.uk (accessed 27 October 2015).

National Institute for Health and Clinical Excellence (NICE) (2012) Caesarean section. *NICE Clinical Guideline 132* (last modified: October 2012). Available online at: www.nice.org.uk (accessed 27 October 2015).

National Institute for Health and Care Excellence (NICE) (2013) *Caesarean Section: Evidence Update March 2013*. Available from www.nice.org.uk (accessed 27 October 2015).

Passmore, H. (2014) Obstetric assessment, in Abbott, H., Braithwaite, W. and Ranson, M. (eds) (2014) *Clinical Examination Skills for Healthcare Professionals*. Keswick: M&K Publishing.

Rang, H.P., Dale, M.M., Ritter, J.M., Flower, R.J. and Henderson, G. (2011) *Rang and Dale's Pharmacology* (7th edn). London: Churchill Livingstone.

Royal College of Nursing (RCN) (2005) Perioperative fasting in adults and children. Available online at: www.rcn.org.uk/__data/assets/pdf_file/0009/78678/002800.pdf (accessed 17 September 2014).

Sands (2014) Teardrop stickers. Available online at: www.uk-sands.org/professionals/resources-for-health-professionals/teardrop-stickers (accessed 13 September 2014).

Shields, L. and Werder, H. (2002) *Perioperative Nursing*. London: Greenwich Medical Media.

Cataract surgery: the care of Elizabeth Jones

Melanie Leek

INTRODUCTION AND LEARNING OUTCOMES

The term 'cataract' is defined as an opacity of the crystalline lens of the eye (Riordan-Eva and Cunningham, 2011), and may result from age, trauma (for example, a penetrating eye injury) or be drug induced (for example, due to use of steroids), or may be pre-senile (for example, developing early through diabetes); by contrast, secondary cataracts are the result of another primary ocular disease (Bowling, 2015). Cataracts cause mistiness or blurring of vision (either gradually, or over a period of weeks or months), extreme sensitivity to bright light, reduced colour vision, ghosting of images, double vision or a shadow in the field of vision. An optician will initially diagnose patients as part of routine eye examinations, and will refer the patient directly to a hospital ophthalmologist; this demonstrates an alternative route of referral to many of the other cases in this text.

Cataract surgery is a common procedure in ophthalmic surgery and this case study will explore the patient journey throughout this procedure.

By the end of this case study you will be able to:

- discuss the causes, symptoms and diagnosis of cataract
- explain the sub-Tenon's anaesthetic block technique
- explain the surgical procedure of phacoemulsification of cataract and prosthetic intraocular lens implant
- discuss the patient journey, including the pre-, peri- and postoperative care required during this procedure.

Case outline

Elizabeth Jones is a 71-year-old female who presented with a cataract in her right eye. She has type 2 diabetes and hypertension, and is also suffering from bilateral osteoarthritis of the knees. Following a consultation with the ophthalmologist, Elizabeth was listed for a right phacoemulsification of cataract and insertion of intraocular lens, under local anaesthetic. There are different

---

local anaesthetic techniques used in ophthalmic surgery and Elizabeth was scheduled for a sub-Tenon's block that would be administered by the ophthalmic consultant surgeon performing the surgery. Elizabeth was scheduled for her procedure in the Ophthalmic Day Care Unit, a specialist ophthalmic unit consisting of two operating theatres and a ward area. This unit performs a range of ophthalmic procedures including corneal surgery, squint surgery and oculoplastic surgeries, however cataract surgery is the most common procedure.

Stop and think

What are your initial priorities for Elizabeth's care? What do you think her main concerns may be?

1   **What does the preoperative assessment and preparation process for Elizabeth involve?**

A   Preparation for Elizabeth's surgery commenced approximately two weeks prior to surgery when Elizabeth attended a pre-assessment clinic. She was initially assessed by a nurse who initiated an integrated care pathway (ICP). This included a measurement of her visual acuity (VA); this is the measurement of the acuteness or clearness of central vision. Normal vision is described as 6/6 – meaning at a standard six-metre distance, the subject can read all the letters on the Snellen chart (a chart consisting of graduated letters, symbols or numbers) – and decreases to 6/12, 6/24, etc.

Elizabeth had a biometry reading performed as part of her pre-assessment; this is a reading of the patient's corneal curvature and axial length to determine the dioptre power of their existing lens (Bowling, 2015). This was then reviewed by the operating surgeon to determine the appropriate lens size for implantation; this was recorded in the ICP. Ophthalmic theatres keep a stock of lenses and surgeons are required to inform theatres if they wish to use a lens not kept within this bank. Elizabeth required a 23.5 dioptre lens, which is held in stock as it is a common-sized lens for implantation. Elizabeth also received dilating drops to both eyes; this allows assessment of the extent of pupil dilation for surgery and examination of the retina under the slit lamp. The slit lamp is a diagnostic tool that combines a light and a microscope, and allows examination of the eye, particularly allowing stereoscopic imaging. Due to this pupil dilation, Elizabeth was instructed not to drive to the pre-assessment clinic, and so was accompanied by her daughter both for transport and also to allow pertinent information to be disseminated to all those involved in the pre- and postoperative care, with Elizabeth's consent.

The pre-assessment appointment includes an explanation of the operative process and Elizabeth was given the opportunity to ask questions; this information was reinforced in an information booklet detailing the pre- and postoperative procedures. Elizabeth then consented for surgery at this time, and, as surgeons list their own patients for surgery, she was given an admission date. Elizabeth was given Minims

Cyclopentolate 1% (a midriatic that dilates the pupil and paralyses the cilary muscle) (BNF, 2015), so that dilation of the pupil on the day of surgery can begin at home; consequently patients are discouraged from driving themselves to the unit on the day of surgery, and will require a friend or relative to take them home after surgery.

2 **How will Elizabeth be prepared on the day of her surgery?**

A Once Elizabeth had been admitted to the day unit, more dilating drops were administered; these consisted of three more doses of cyclopentolate 1%, three doses of G. Ocufen and three doses of phenylephrine 2.5% given at 20-minute intervals; these ensure maximum dilation of the pupil and G. Ocufen inhibits intraoperative miosis. Some patients find the administration of these drops painful, and the degree of discomfort will depend on the individual pain threshold – however this does wear off within a few minutes. Elizabeth was also given tetracaine 1% and povidone iodine 5% just prior to collection for surgery. Tetracaine is a local anaesthetic and povidone iodine acts as an antiseptic agent (BNF, 2015).

Elizabeth was dressed for theatre in a theatre gown over her normal clothes, and had been asked to bring her dressing gown and slippers with her; these are worn over the theatre gown. Just before collection for theatre, Elizabeth was advised to visit the toilet and was then helped into the theatre chair, which can be converted into an operating table in the anaesthetic room, ready for the perioperative support worker (PSW) to collect her for theatre.

The PSW who collected Elizabeth checked her details against the theatre list (i.e. name, date of birth and hospital number), and verbally confirmed with her the side of surgery and allergy status. He then explained what was happening and gave her the chance to ask any questions before taking her through to the anaesthetic room.

3 **How would you prepare the theatre environment for the cataract surgery list?**

A Specific theatre preparation for a cataract list involves testing the phacoemulsification machine, and loading settings for the individual surgeon operating, as each surgeon has their own specific settings. The microscope is also tested and placed in the required position.

Irrigation during the surgery is provided by a one-litre bag of balanced salt solution (BSS); this is a solution of sodium chloride, sodium citrate, sodium acetate, calcium chloride and potassium chloride (BNF, 2015), into which is added 0.5 ml of adrenaline 1:1000; adrenaline is added to maintain dilation of the pupil during surgery. All the required drugs and fluids for surgery are made available; these include Betadine antiseptic, sterile water, cefuroxime, adrenaline, gentamicin, BSS and viscoelastic.

There are also specific records that are kept for ophthalmic surgery; these include a lens order sheet, an intraocular drug record and a lens register. Records are kept of the lot number and expiry dates of intraocular drugs so that, should the patient develop complications related to drugs, the particular batch can be traced.

4 **How was the surgical site marked?**

A The side of surgery was verbally confirmed, as were Elizabeth's details against the theatre list and the ICP. At this time the side of the operation was marked with a surgical marker pen to draw an arrow over the eye to be operated on; the mark is removed at the completion of surgery by rubbing it with a damp swab. This is to prevent wrong-site surgery and complies with the Royal College of Ophthalmologists' *Cataract Surgery Guidelines* (2010). At this time the 'sign in' section of the Surgical Safety Checklist can be completed.

5   **What anaesthetic techniques are considered for cataract surgery and why?**

A   The majority of patients having cataract surgery will have a local anaesthetic, but a general anaesthetic may be considered – for example, for a patient who has Parkinson's disease and who may not be able to keep their head still enough for surgery – and some patients may be offered intravenous sedation – for example, those who are extremely nervous.

6   **How is a sub-Tenon's block administered?**

A   Elizabeth had her surgery under local anaesthetic, in this case a sub-Tenon's block. This is a proven technique that offers a high degree of akinesia (the absence or impairment of voluntary movement) and analgesia, which is important for intraoperative and postoperative pain relief. Some surgeons perform cataract surgery using only topical anaesthesia, and while this is a quicker technique that avoids the potential complications related to sub-Tenon's block, it does not provide any akinesia. Under topical anaesthesia therefore the patient is still able to move their eye in any direction and they may do so at any time; if this happens at a particularly delicate moment surgical complications may occur – for example, a dropped nucleus when the posterior capsule is breached, and part or all of the nucleus may fall into the vitreous cavity. If this occurs, referral to a vitreoretinal surgeon is required and more extensive surgery will be required to remove the fragment (Sundaram *et al.*, 2009).

In order for the block to be administered, the patient must be in a supine position and this is maintained for the duration of the surgery. As Elizabeth has osteoarthritis in her knees she was made more comfortable by putting a pillow under her knees. The block was administered by the surgeon, and involved using a sub-Tenon's cannula to insert a volume of local anaesthetic into the sub-Tenon's fascia space. A sub-Tenon's cannula differs from other cannulas in that it is blunt ended and slightly curved so that it can be passed around the globe of the eye easily. For Elizabeth's block, a cannula 25 mm long and 19G was used. Anaesthesia of the conjunctiva was first achieved by the drop of 1% tetracaine, a small incision was then made into the conjunctiva approximately 10 mm from the limbus in the infero-nasal region. The cannula on a loaded syringe was passed into the potential space following the curve of the globe, usually to a depth of 1.5–2 cm; akinesia, analgesia and hypotonia are achieved a few minutes following administration. Common complications related to the sub-Tenon's technique are chemosis and haemorrhage (McLeod, McCartney and Wildsmith, 2012), however it is also important to be aware of the risk of misplacement of the needle and the subsequent complications (Hadzic, 2007). The choice of anaesthetic drug and the volume of anaesthetic solution used varies between different surgeons, and could be 1% or 2% lignocaine with or without adrenaline, 0.5% Marcain®, 2% or 4% articaine, 1% ropivacaine, 0.75% levobupivacaine or 2% mepivacaine, and the volume can vary from 1 to 11 ml. The addition of Hyalase® – an enzyme that enhances the infiltration and dispersal of the anaesthetic into the ocular tissues – is again according to the surgeon's preference as there is the risk of an allergic reaction to Hyalase® and, although this is rare, it can cause swelling, itchiness, gross conjunctival chemosis, pain or decreased vision (Leek, 2011).

Elizabeth's sub-Tenon's block was a combination of 5 ml 2% lignocaine with adrenaline 1:200,000, plus 75 IU/ml Hyalase®. If the patient has a known allergy to Hyalase® this will be omitted. Following administration of the anaesthetic, a further drop of 5% povidone iodine was placed in the eye. When sufficient akinesia had been achieved – this was assessed by asking the Elizabeth to look up, down, left and right – Elizabeth was taken through to the operating theatre, where a pulse oximetry probe was placed, and a bar fixed on to the operating table to keep the surgical drape from lying on Elizabeth's face and keep it away from her nose and mouth.

7 **How should Elizabeth be monitored and supported during her surgery?**

A During surgery all patients have their pulse and oxygen saturations monitored, and recorded in the ICP. The Royal College of Ophthalmologists' guidelines (2010) state that a practitioner trained to detect and act on adverse events should be responsible for monitoring the patient; this may be an operating department practitioner or anaesthetic nurse who has undertaken the Immediate Life Support course.

Verbal communication during surgery is discouraged, as talking will result in some movement of the patient's head, and therefore their eye. As Elizabeth was to remain awake for her surgery it is important that communication was still maintained between her and the theatre team; this was achieved by asking Elizabeth to raise her hand if she needed the surgery to stop for any reason, such as wanting to cough, sneeze or move in any way, or if she is experiencing any pain. Some patients may wish to hold the hand of one of the theatre team and then they can squeeze if they wish the surgery to be halted; hand holding can also provide psychological support and comfort for the patient. Many patients find the human contact provided by a hand holder to be reassuring and comforting (Mitchell, 2008), but others may feel uncomfortable holding a stranger's hand, and so to individualise each patient's operative experience they are asked if they would like a hand to hold (Mokashi et al., 2004). Elizabeth opted to have a hand holder, and this was done by the PSW. Perioperative staff acting as a 'hand holder' for ophthalmic surgery must be aware that their movements may transfer to the patient and cause movement of the eye.

8 **Prior to commencement of surgery, what process is undertaken to reduce the risk of error?**

A Before commencement of the surgery the 'time out' section of the Surgical Safety Checklist was completed. This involved verbally confirming with the surgeon, scrub practitioner, circulator and anaesthetic practitioner the patient's name, allergy status, side the surgery is to be performed and the dioptre size of the lens to be inserted. These details were written on a whiteboard in theatre too, for reference during surgery. If any additional equipment is required – for example, iris hooks, capsular tension ring or an anterior chamber lens – this is also recorded on the whiteboard. The Surgical Safety Checklist used for Elizabeth had been adapted locally from the document produced by the National Patient Safety Agency (NPSA) (2010), and is used specifically in ophthalmology theatres to avoid 'never events' such as the wrong operation on the correct eye, or the correct operation on the wrong eye (NPSA, 2009).

q **How will Elizabeth's surgery be performed?**

A Once Elizabeth was settled in the theatre the operative area was prepped with aqueous povidone iodine solution and an ophthalmic drape placed over her eye by the surgeon; a hole was cut into this to enable the speculum to be placed. Elizabeth's other eye was taped closed prior to positioning of the drape, which helps to prevent blinking. The cornea is kept hydrated with balanced salt solution during surgery to prevent corneal injury and maintain the surgeon's view by preventing clouding of the cornea.

The surgical team had prepared the specialised equipment required for this operation, primarily a phacoemulsification machine and handpiece. Several manufacturers make these machines, each using their own specific disposables. A basic intraocular tray was used, which in the current practice area consists of forceps, scissors, needle holders, a speculum and a lens manipulator that, due to its shape at the end, is called a 'mushroom'. This combination of instruments is specific to this ophthalmic unit and will vary from hospital to hospital, but these individual instruments will be found in most ophthalmic theatres.

Elizabeth had her cataract removed using the phacoemulsification technique. Phacoemulsification is the disassembly and removal of the crystalline lens and is described by Bowling (2015) and Sundaram et al. (2009) in the following stages.

- A self-sealing tunnel incision (less than 3 mm wide) was made into the anterior chamber, and a viscoelastic substance injected into it – the viscoelastic substance is a transparent viscous gel, and is used to stabilise the anterior chamber and maintain its depth before the capsulorhexis is performed. This also protects the corneal endothelium from mechanical trauma and ultrasound energy during phacoemulsification.
- Second stab incisions are made at right angles to the first. A capsulorhexis (a circular hole in the anterior capsule) is performed and hydro dissection performed (BSS is gently injected) to mobilise the nucleus. Using a hand-held ultrasonic vibrator, a groove is sculpted into the nucleus, which is rotated, and a second groove made at right angles to the first. The nucleus is cracked into four segments at the base of the groove. Each quadrant is fragmented, emulsified and aspirated.
- The remaining cortex is aspirated and more viscoelastic substance added to inflate the capsular bag into which the foldable lens is injected. The remaining viscoelastic substance is removed and, as the wound is self-sealing, no sutures are required. This method avoids sutures, and gives rapid wound healing and reduced postoperative inflammation, all of which improve visual rehabilitation (Riordan-Eva and Cunningham, 2011).

At the end of surgery all patients will receive a prophylactic dose of antibiotics. Should the patient be allergic to penicillin, gentamycin is given, but in Elizabeth's case, as no such allergy existed she was given a dose of intracameral cefuroxime. After completion of surgery as described above, the drape was removed, the povidone iodine and surgical site mark cleaned off the skin, and a dressing of a folded 10 cm x 10 cm paraffin gauze placed over the closed eye. An eye pad and clear plastic shield were taped into position with micropore tape. The 'sign out' section of the Surgical Safety Checklist was completed, the operation notes in the ICP completed by the surgeon, and an optician postoperative referral form completed.

10   **What postoperative care did Elizabeth require in the ophthalmic day care unit?**

A   Elizabeth was returned to the ward area, and after transferring her from the theatre chair to a normal ward chair, a handover was given by the ODP to the ward nurse caring for her. This involved a confirmation of the patient's name and the procedure performed, and specific outpatient requirements, and any untoward incidents there may have been during surgery (none in Elizabeth's case). Patients who have no additional ophthalmic conditions to their cataract will routinely go to their own optician for postoperative assessment. Basic observations were taken on Elizabeth's return, including her blood pressure and heart rate. Elizabeth was given a cup of tea and, as she was diabetic, some plain biscuits, while the postoperative to-take-away (TTA) drops were dispensed; Elizabeth had been prescribed a one-month course of Maxitrol – a mix of dexamethasone, neomycin and polymyxin B sulphate – used for the short-term treatment of inflammation, three times daily (BNF, 2015). Explanations were given to Elizabeth and her daughter of how to administer the drops, and contact numbers given in case of adverse events such as pain, inflammation of the eye and surrounding tissues, or a sudden loss of vision. The sub-Tenon's block should provide immediate postoperative pain relief, and last for three to four hours. As the anaesthetic wears off and muscle movement is regained, it is quite common for patients to experience some double vision. Some blurred vision may also occur; this again will clear as the effects of the anaesthetic wear off. Elizabeth is not a driver, but those patients who are, are advised not to drive until there are no residual effects of the anaesthetic, and may do so only if the ophthalmologist has given permission prior to surgery.

The use of the clear plastic shield was explained to Elizabeth, who was told to remove the dressing the next morning but keep the shield to wear overnight for one week, to prevent inadvertent injury to the eye by rubbing in the night. After getting changed, Elizabeth was escorted home by her daughter, who stayed with her that night; it is not vital that patients have someone stay with them overnight after their surgery, but some may benefit from the security of a friend or relative staying with them, particularly elderly patients.

REFERENCES AND FURTHER READING

Bowling, B. (2015) *Kanski's Clinical Ophthalmology: A Systematic Approach* (8th edn). Edinburgh: Elsevier Health Sciences Ltd.

British National Formulary (BNF) (2015) *BNF 70*. London: BMJ Publishing Group Ltd/RPS Publishing.

Hadzic, A. (ed.) (2007) *Textbook of Regional Anaesthesia and Acute Pain Management*. New York: McGraw-Hill Medical.

Leek, M. (2011) Sub-Tenon's drug combination and volume: a systematic review, *Technic: The Journal of Operating Department Practice*, **2**(1): 10–13.

McLeod, G., McCartney, C. and Wildsmith, T. (2012) *Principles and Practice of Regional Anaesthesia* (4th edn). Oxford: Oxford University Press.

Mitchell, M. (2008) Conscious surgery: influence of the environment on patient anxiety. *Journal of Advanced Nursing*, **62**(3): 261–271.

Mokashi, A., Leatherbarrow, B., Kinsey, J., Slater, R., Hillier, V. and Mayer, S. (2004) Patient communication during cataract surgery. *Eye*, **18**: 147–151.

National Patient Safety Agency (NPSA) (2009) Never Events Framework 2009/10. Available online at: www.nrls.npsa.nhs.uk/neverevents (accessed 4 March 2014).

National Patient Safety Agency (NPSA) (2010) WHO Surgical Safety Checklist: for cataract surgery only. Available online at: www.nrls.npsa.nhs.ik/resources/clinical-speciality/ophthalmology/?entryid45=74132 (accessed 4 March 2014).

Riordan-Eva, P. and Cunningham, E.T. (eds) (2011) *Vaughn and Asbury's General Ophthalmology* (18th edn). New York: McGraw-Hill Medical.

Royal College of Ophthalmologists (2010) *Cataract Surgery Guidelines*. London: RCO.

Sundaram, V., Barsam, A., Alwitry, A. and Khaw, P.T. (eds) (2009) *Training in Ophthalmology*. New York: Oxford University Press.

Cleft palate and myringotomy: the care of Ronnie Bass

Ray Swann

INTRODUCTION AND LEARNING OUTCOMES

Cleft lip and palate is a congenital abnormality resulting in incomplete fusion of the lip and palate during gestation, and occurs to varying degrees in approximately 1 in 700 live births (Hupp, Ellis and Tucker, 2014). The lip and palate deformities may be physically disfiguring with a potential negative impact on functionality in terms of mastication, swallowing, speech and hearing, and therefore treatment requires a broad approach involving a multidisciplinary team.

By the end of this case study you will be able to:

- understand the need for a multidisciplinary team approach in caring for a child born with a cleft lip and palate
- understand the patient's and parental needs when managing cleft lip and palate repair
- understand key considerations in the anaesthetic, surgical and post-anaesthetic care management of a child undergoing a cleft palate repair.

Case outline

Ronnie Bass is a 12-month-old boy born with a unilateral cleft lip and palate defect. The cleft defect in Ronnie's case additionally resulted in abnormal insertion of the muscles (Hupp *et al.*, 2014) that facilitate opening of the eustachian tube into the nasopharynx, resulting in reduced drainage of serous fluid from the middle ear and potential for otitis media. If chronic infection develops there is the possibility of subsequent hearing impairment, hence the need for myringotomy and insertion of grommets simultaneously with the palate repair.

Repair of cleft lip and palate can be a multi-stage process commencing shortly after birth and into teenage years dependent upon severity, growth and anatomical development. Early repair of the cleft lip helps reduce parental anxiety resulting from the physical disfigurement but also helps improve feeding as, without this, suckling and maintaining an effective seal is difficult.

Ronnie had his cleft lip repaired at three months under general anaesthetic with no complications. Planned palate repair at seven months was delayed due to an upper respiratory tract infection. On presenting for surgery at 12 months he was generally fit and well.

1   **It is important that a number of different practitioners are included within the preoperative preparation process for Ronnie. Who do you think these are and what are their roles?**

A   The complex nature of cleft lip and palate surgery requires a multidisciplinary team (MDT) approach, including but not limited to specialist nurses, and plastic, maxillofacial and ENT surgeons, anaesthetists, orthodontists, speech and language therapists, audiologists and clinical psychologists. Prior to surgery Ronnie had a full review by the MDT and the long-term potential treatment options were discussed with his parents.

In addition to the MDT, Shields (2010) recognises the important role of partnership between parents and health professionals in the provision of care for the hospitalised child, and Ronnie and his parents attended a preoperative assessment clinic two weeks prior to surgery. His parents received full verbal and supporting written information on the planned surgery and anaesthetic, including possible adverse outcomes, to allow an informed decision on which to give their consent and ask questions (Royal College of Anaesthetists (RCoA), 2015).

Parental presence in the anaesthetic room is generally advocated in the UK to help reduce children's anxiety. Ronnie's parents were advised that they may accompany him to theatre, and what to expect during induction and postoperatively in the post-anaesthetic care unit (PACU). In addition to caring for the child, it is essential that the perioperative practitioner recognises the potential for heightened parental anxiety during the perioperative 'journey' and responds compassionately to their emotional needs, providing reassurance and effective communication as required.

2   **What do you think the key components of Ronnie's anaesthetic assessment and preparation include?**

A   Anaesthetic assessment included complete birth and medical history and assessment of the cardiovascular system and airway, including baseline observations (Table 10.1). Cleft palate is associated with a number of other potential syndromes that can adversely affect the airway (James and Walker, 2013), and pre-assessment considers the extent of any co-morbidities, however none was evident in this case. A review of previous anaesthetic history and that of the family is essential in minimising risk, and Ronnie's previous general anaesthetic at three months was free of complications and provided an indicator for planning the cleft repair.

Weighing of children is extremely important for the calculation of drug dosages and, although in emergency circumstances an estimation of the weight is possible, the ideal for planned surgery is accurate measurement preoperatively. Ronnie was weighed on admission.

Preoperative fasting is advocated, however it is recognised that extended periods of starvation are potentially harmful. Ronnie had started weaning on puréed solids

Table 10.1 Summary of baseline observations for Ronnie

	Normal range	Actual
Weight (kg)		9
Pulse rate (beats/minute)	80–120	105
Blood pressure (mmHg)	(95–110)/(55–70)	107/70
Respiratory rate (breaths/minute)	20–30	30
Temperature (degrees Celsius)	36–38	36

Source: Doyle (2007)

supplemented by bottle feeding on formula milk. Fasting was required from six hours preoperatively for solids and formula milk, however clear fluids were encouraged and provided until two hours preoperatively (James and Walker, 2013).

Although excessive blood loss was not envisaged with cleft palate repair, blood samples were taken during the pre-assessment, providing a baseline haemoglobin measurement and allowing one unit to be grouped and saved (Doyle, 2007).

3 **How would you prepare the theatre environment and theatre team for this case?**

A Caring for children in the perioperative environment requires the whole perioperative team to fully recognise that individuals in their care are not just small adults, and that altered physiological and anatomical development – allied with distinct emotional needs – present very specific challenges. There is an expectation that all staff involved in the perioperative care have specific training in order to safely and effectively manage this patient group (RCoA, 2015).

The RCoA (2015) advocates that a full range of equipment suitable for use with babies and children should be available wherever they are anesthetised or recovered. A summary of these recommendations is provided here:

- airway management and monitoring equipment, including capnography and difficult airway management equipment
- paediatric oximetry sensors and blood pressure cuffs
- vascular access equipment, including intraosseous needles
- burettes and syringe pumps to allow rapid and accurate fluid and drug delivery
- fluid and external warming devices
- resuscitation drugs, equipment and appropriate defibrillator
- anaesthetic machine incorporating ventilators, with flexibility to be used over full age range, and with accurate pressure control and PEEP (Positive End Expiratory Pressure)
- thermostatic control of the theatre up to 26–28 degrees Celsius.

The shared airway between the anaesthetist and surgeon in this case presents challenges in, for example, airway compromise and surgical access which is further complicated by the use of an operating microscope. To help alleviate this issue the operating table was turned 180 degrees with the anaesthetic machine distal to the head.

Specialist instrumentation is a prerequisite in all surgical areas, and in this case included aural instrumentation, instrumentation to facilitate access and surgery on the palate, and an operating microscope as a minimum requirement. The list below is not definitive and local requirements should always be considered, but it provides some examples of specialist equipment that may be needed:

- aural instrumentation – speculum, probes, myringotomes, crocodile forceps
- oral instrumentation – mouth gag and rods, BP handles and blades, beaver blades, angled scissors, elevators, needle holders, long dissecting forceps, bipolar diathermy.

The perioperative team ensured availability and serviceability of all anaesthetic and surgical equipment prior to commencing the operating list; this was confirmed at the preoperative team brief.

4   **How would you care for Ronnie to ensure safe induction of anaesthesia?**

A   Ronnie was escorted to theatre by a registered children's nurse and his mother, with the perioperative practitioner. Induction is a potentially traumatic time for children and parents, and although having been briefed preoperatively Ronnie's mother was clearly upset. To reduce her anxiety, the perioperative practitioner provided both commentary on what was happening and reassurance that involuntary twitching, noisy breathing and Ronnie 'going limp' were indeed normal at induction of anaesthesia.

Cannulation and application of monitoring before induction, although preferable, may cause excessive pain and emotional distress in children, therefore it was decided to induce Ronnie rapidly using inhalational induction, and only a paediatric pulse oximetry probe was applied initially.

Inhalational induction using sevoflurane in 100% oxygen via a low dead space face mask and T-piece circuit allowed spontaneous ventilation to be maintained and the airway to be assessed prior to muscle relaxation and assisted ventilation. Sevoflurane was chosen for induction and subsequent maintenance due to its rapid onset, non-irritant nature, and its facilitation of rapid emergence and recovery (Paediatric Formulary Committee, 2015). Following induction full monitoring was applied and temperature monitoring was achieved via a rectal probe given the issues of shared airway. Intravenous access was secured using a 22G cannula and IV drug administration commenced on confirmation that the airway could be maintained via face mask. Table 10.2 provides a summary of perioperative pharmacological interventions.

5   **What are the anatomical differences that will impact upon the management of Ronnie's airway? How would you prepare for these?**

A   James and Walker (2013) recognise that anatomical differences in small children, such as relatively large tongue and epiglottis, require a different approach to laryngoscopy and endotracheal (ET) intubation, and this is further complicated when a cleft deformity is present. A straight-blade laryngoscope can help improve visualisation during laryngoscopy with small children and this was used to intubate Ronnie with

Table 10.2 Pharmacological interventions during anaesthesia

Drugs	Rationale
Remifentanil	Short-acting synthetic opioid – reduces volatile agent requirements and helps promote rapid emergence
Atracurium	Non-depolarising muscle relaxant to facilitate endotracheal intubation and IPPV
Bupivacaine 0.25% with 1:200,000 adrenaline	Analgesia and haemostasis to reduce blood loss and improve the surgical field
Analgesia – morphine and paracetamol	Intravenous multimodal approach to analgesia to ensure comfort, and reduce agitation and crying on emergence
Cefuroxime	Intravenous antibiotic prophylaxis
Dexamethasone	Anti-emetic and reduces oedema

Sources: Paediatric Formulary Committee (2015); Doyle (2007)

a south-facing size 4 uncuffed RAE tube. Intermittent positive pressure ventilation (IPPV) was maintained throughout the procedure.

Prior to extubation, nasopharyngeal airways were inserted by the surgeon to help maintain a patent airway postoperatively and additionally providing a route for gentle suctioning of the oral pharyngeal space while reducing potential trauma to the surgical site (James and Walker, 2013). Ronnie was extubated in the operating theatre by the anaesthetist once all protective reflexes had returned, and then transferred to the paediatric post-anaesthetic care unit (PPACU) with 100% supplemental oxygen.

6   **The myringotomy is performed first, what does this involve?**

A   Ronnie was initially positioned supine on the operating table with a head ring in place for stabilisation during the myringotomies (Doyle, 2007). Myringotomy involves a small incision in the tympanic membrane under microscopy using a myringotome, followed by insertion of a tympanostomy tube or grommet.

7   **How is the repair of the cleft palate performed?**

A   Ronnie was repositioned following myringotomy with a small gel bolster under his shoulders to extend the neck and facilitate improved access to the operative site. Repair of the palatal defect in a small child is complicated by limited access and relatively limited vision, and the use of a split mouth gag and rods maintained the mouth open while helping prevent movement of the ET tube.

Hupp *et al.* (2014) recognise that each cleft lip and palate is unique with variances in, for example, defect width, extent of hard and soft palate involved, and palatal length. It is therefore indicative that techniques for surgical repair vary widely, however the key objectives remain the same: separating the oral and nasal cavities and, in doing so, allowing a mechanism for effective swallowing and speech development while facilitating further maxillary and dental growth. The perioperative scrub practitioner should understand the generic principles underlying palatal repair while remaining responsive and flexible to the individual surgical demands.

Ronnie had initial infiltration of the palate using bupivacaine 0.25% with adrenaline 1:200,000, and additional haemostasis was achieved using a combination of bipolar diathermy and pressure using 'tonsil' swabs. Repair of the palatal cleft was performed with the aid of the operating microscope, and involved lateral incisions and dissection along the cleft margins using a combination of scissors, blades and specialist elevators to free tissue. Opposing edges were then approximated and sutured thereby closing the defect and lengthening the palate. Closure was in three layers using 5/0 Vicryl in the following order: nasal mucosa, muscle, oral mucosa.

8   How will Ronnie's intraoperative homeostasis be maintained?

A   The avoidance of inadvertent perioperative hypothermia is an important consideration in all patients, with children being particularly prone to a reduction in core temperature (Doyle, 2007), therefore monitoring and actions to reduce the occurrence are essential. In this case the ambient theatre temperature was raised from 21 to 23 degrees Celsius. Forced air warming and the use of heat and moisture exchange filters on the breathing circuit also contributed to the maintenance of normothermia. Anticipated and actual blood loss was relatively small for the procedure, however the administration of maintenance fluids was advocated given the period of fasting combined with the duration of surgery (approximately one and a half to two hours). A bolus of Hartmann's solution was given perioperatively with the aid of a volumetric pump and a counter-current warming system, which additionally helped in maintaining normothermia.

9   What do you need to consider when caring for Ronnie in the PPACU?

A   The post-anaesthetic care unit (PACU) has a designated area for recovering children that is separate from the adult area and child friendly in terms of decor. This area – the paediatric post-anaesthetic care unit (PPACU) – is specially equipped for dealing with children and potential clinical emergencies in this patient group, as recommended by the Royal College of Anaesthetists (2015).

The recovery practitioner provided one-to-one care, ensuring close monitoring and supervision as children can regain consciousness quickly following anaesthesia. Recognising the potential for sudden rapid movement combined with the use of padded cot sides helped to reduce the risk of Ronnie receiving an unintentional physical injury. Postoperative observations were recorded every 15 minutes using a paediatric early warning score (PEWS) chart, which continued on the ward following transfer for a minimum of two hours and included the following:

- heart rate/pulse
- respiratory rate
- respiratory distress
- blood pressure
- pulse oximetry for oxygen saturation
- any oxygen being administered

- any nurse/doctor or family concern
- any decreases in conscious level or new irritability
- temperature.

Monitoring of the airway is essential in this patient group, with surgical site bleeding, oedema and swelling of the tongue following compression with the mouth gag being potential causes of airway compromise. Adequate oxygen saturation without supplemental oxygen was a prerequisite before transfer to the ward, and Ronnie's immediate postoperative care – with the exception of additional analgesia being administered – was uneventful.

Anxiety and crying may increase the likelihood of postoperative bleeding (Doyle, 2007), therefore controlling pain and providing emotional support are essential postoperatively. A number of tools are available for assessing and scoring pain in children (Shields, 2010) with FLACC (face, legs, activity, cry and consolability) being the tool of choice in the unit described here. The multimodal approach to analgesia continued postoperatively, with an additional bolus of morphine IV being administered in response to the FLACC score. Continuing prescribed analgesia included paracetamol and ibuprofen (orally) four times daily, with oral morphine as required.

Ronnie's mother and a registered paediatric nurse attended the recovery area within 15 minutes of Ronnie's arrival; this was a key factor in reducing his anxiety. Full handover to the ward staff included all observations and a summary of surgical and anaesthetic interventions, including prescribed analgesia and the indwelling nasopharygeal airways that would be removed following a medical review on the ward.

10 **What ongoing care and review do you think Ronnie may require?**

A Correction of cleft deformities, as indicated earlier, can be a prolonged process into teenage years and although the prognosis in terms of physical appearance and functionality may be good, the continued input of the multidisciplinary team and support for the patient and parents are essential. Ronnie's ongoing management by the cleft team will include reviews by audiologists, speech and language therapists, and the dental team that in turn dictate the need for further surgery where in specialised units the perioperative staff may see patients returning several times as they mature.

Stop and think

Having read this case study, you will have seen that there are a number of considerations when caring for Ronnie. Reflect upon your own experiences of managing more complex cases and consider how confident you feel in this aspect of perioperative care. You should try to identify areas where you feel you could improve further and how you might achieve this.

REFERENCES AND FURTHER READING

Doyle, E. (2007) *Paediatric Anaesthesia.* Oxford: Oxford University Press.

Goldenberg, D. and Goldstein, B.J. (2011) *Handbook of Otolaryngology – Head and Neck Surgery.* New York: Thieme Medical Publishers.

Hupp, J.R., Ellis III, E. and Tucker, M.R. (2014) *Contemporary Oral and Maxillofacial Surgery* (6th edn). St Louis, MO: Mosby Elsevier.

James, I. and Walker, I. (2013) *Core Topics in Paediatric Anaesthesia.* Cambridge: Cambridge University Press.

Kaban, L.B. and Trouis, M.J. (2004) *Pediatric Oral and Maxillofacial Surgery.* Philadelphia: Saunders (an imprint of Elsevier).

Miloro, M. and Kolokythas, A. (2012) *Management of Complications in Oral and Maxillofacial Surgery.* Chichester: Wiley Blackwell.

Paediatric Formulary Committee (2015) *BNF for Children.* London: Pharmaceutical Press.

Royal College of Anaesthetists (RCoA) (2015) Guidelines for the provision of anaesthetic services: paediatric anaesthesia services 2014. Available online at: www.rcoa.ac.uk/system/files/GPAS-2015–10-PAEDIATRICS.pdf (accessed 18 September 2015).

Shields, L. (2010) *Perioperative Care of the Child: A Nursing Manual.* Chichester: Wiley-Blackwell.

CASE STUDY 11

Flexible bronchoscopy: the care of Spiros Papandrea

Stephen Wordsworth

INTRODUCTION AND LEARNING OUTCOMES

This case study details the perioperative care of a patient undergoing a diagnostic bronchoscopy. In recent years the use of bronchoscopy has been significantly enhanced due to rapid advances in technology such that it is now a widely used technique with a number of applications; these range from diagnostic or investigative procedures through to various imaging techniques, biopsy and therapeutic interventions.

By the end of this case study you will be able to:

- describe the pre-, peri- and postoperative care needs of the patient undergoing bronchoscopy
- establish the rationale for bronchoscopy, and the benefits and drawbacks to the procedure from the patient's perspective
- explain the technique of bronchoscopy, and its safe and effective use.

Case outline

Spiros Papandrea is 55 years old and a British-born second-generation Greek Cypriot. He lives with his wife and two children in their family home. Spiros and his wife were married in their mid-twenties and had their first child, a daughter, two years after that. Spiros has always worked in the printing industry, working his way up through several promotions before becoming the area manager responsible for the day-to-day running of a print factory. In his early thirties he started his own printing business and has been working hard putting in long days to make this the success that it is today. Their second child was born when Spiros and his wife were in their late thirties.

While spending some rare quality time playing football with his children, Spiros first noticed how quickly he became out of breath. Spiros has been a smoker for all of his adult life, and both of his children had encouraged Spiros to stop smoking, noticing how much longer it took their dad to 'get his breath back'. A number of years earlier Spiros had to take some time off work because

---

of exhaustion, and made the excuse that he was 'just run down again', and that he felt he probably needed a holiday. His wife, however, was not convinced and pointed out that Spiros had developed a persistent cough; she urged him to do something about it.

Spiros presented to his GP two weeks later; he described episodes of breathlessness and said that he generally felt more tired and lethargic than he would normally. Otherwise he reported being fit and well. In terms of lifestyle, Spiros drinks alcohol only occasionally and not in excess of the recommended 21 units per week. Although he has cut down the number of cigarettes he smokes, this is still around 15 per day. He does not exercise particularly but is not overweight and would appear to have a normal body mass index (BMI) for someone of average height. A detailed family history reveals no evidence of stroke, however his father died from a heart attack and his paternal grandfather was diagnosed with lung cancer. When asked about his eating habits, Spiros suggested that he 'didn't have much of an appetite', which he joked was 'down to his and his wife's bad cooking, and his busy work life'. Spiros indicated that he did not have any allergies and that he was not currently taking any medication. The GP confirmed that baseline observations – temperature, pulse and BP – were normal. Heart sounds were also normal, with no obvious tenderness to the chest wall. Auscultation of the patient's breath sounds did not reveal any obvious abnormalities.

1 **What is the aetiology and the clinical symptoms that suggest the need for Spiros to undergo bronchoscopy?**

A The GP was concerned about the episode of breathlessness (dyspnoea) in conjunction with co-morbidities such as a cough that had appeared in the absence of any other signs of a cold and chest infection. Possible familial predisposition to lung cancer alone indicates that susceptibility is increased three-fold compared to the general population (Cancer Care UK, 2016). The risk of developing lung cancer is also dependent upon the patient's age, the number of cigarettes smoked, the duration of smoking (in years), the degree of inhalation, and the tar and nicotine content of the particular brand of cigarette (Cancer Care UK, 2016).

Stop and think

In addition to the presence of a persistent cough, what other clinical symptoms could also indicate the possibility of lung cancer?

- Haemoptysis (bleeding)

As well as any of the following unexplained or persistent symptoms (more than three weeks):

- cough
- chest and or shoulder pain

- dyspnoea
- weight loss
- chest signs
- hoarseness
- finger clubbing
- features suggestive of metastasis
- cervical/supraclavicular lymphadenopathy.

Source: NICE Clinical Guideline 121 (2011)

Although Spiros suggested that he felt he had developed his cough 'a few weeks ago', his wife, who had accompanied him to the GP, felt that he had been coughing for more like a month. This kind of unexplained chronic cough that persists for more than three weeks again alerted the GP to the presence of possible bronchogenic carcinoma (NICE, 2011). This alone however is not conclusive evidence and could indicate a number of other possible causes, including the presence of aggravants such as asthma, drug inhalation, environmental factors, gastro-oesophageal reflux, the presence of a foreign body, and a number of other pathologies or indeed infections (Morice, McGarvey and Pavord, 2006).

2 **Which other investigative procedures should be included in Spiros's diagnostic pathway?**

A A chest x-ray was requested to aid diagnosis, but internal organs such as the heart and aorta can hide significantly enlarged areas of lung tissue, therefore an x-ray alone cannot confirm the difference between a bronchogenic carcinoma or a benign granuloma, and even the latter is not thought to be visible until it is 2–3 cm in size (Du Rand *et al.*, 2013). In this case nothing definitive was found and in such cases of occult radiography, the next stage would be to perform a chest computed tomography (CT) scan to find the extent and spread of a possible tumour. On CT Spiros was found to have a single central hilar mass in the region of the right superior lobar bronchus. The lesion appeared well defined at 1.5 cm in diameter, with no obvious signs of spreading to surrounding tissue or lymph nodes.

In Spiros's case the next step is to perform a bronchoscopy. Along with CT this forms an important step in the diagnostic pathway.

3 **Discuss the psychological preparation of a patient undergoing diagnostic bronchoscopy for possible carcinoma.**

A A number of initial stages were undertaken to prepare Spiros for bronchoscopy, from a technical viewpoint and – given the potential psychological impact of the potential diagnosis – to help him to address the emotional aspects of the procedure. At his initial consultation with his GP, Spiros had been reluctant to talk about his symptoms, but after receiving the results of his x-ray, he began to ask his GP about his likely diagnosis and outcome. In line with NICE (2011) best practice guidelines, his GP was keen that Spiros should be able to make informed decisions in partnership with a range of healthcare professionals. Patient-centred care such as this also encourages the patient to involve other family members, and Spiros was keen for his wife to be as informed and involved as he was.

Because the chest x-ray appeared normal despite the suspicion of lung cancer, Spiros was offered the opportunity for referral to a member of the lung cancer team, in this case a specialist chest physician. Initially he decided to wait until the outcome of the CT scan, but following receipt of the results met with his consultant physician. Although the diagnosis was not conclusive, Spiros was informed it was highly likely to be a carcinoma but at this stage it was not possible to be specific about the type. However, his consultant was encouraged that the tumour had been detected at a very early stage, which is always an important factor in treating the disease.

Although Spiros was naturally shocked by the news, and at first didn't believe what he was hearing, at subsequent meetings he did feel a little less traumatised once his management plan had been discussed with him. Both Spiros and his wife also took advantage of meeting with a lung cancer clinical nurse specialist, at first to speak about Spiros's smoking cessation, but then to help him explore and deal with the emotional outcome of his diagnosis. The clinical nurse specialist was also able to explain how she could facilitate good communication between the various strands of the multidisciplinary team (MDT) and how she could help Spiros access further advice and support, as well as make sure he was involved in his own care and treatment.

4   **Outline the steps taken in Spiros's preoperative preparation.**

A   The procedure of bronchoscopy itself is now acknowledged as an important diagnostic tool, and considered appropriate to undertake in a number of clinical settings. It is generally well tolerated by the patient and is considered a safe procedure, with serious complications occurring in only 1.1% of patients and a mortality rate of 0.02% (Du Rand et al., 2013).

As part of the normal preoperative preparation Spiros was provided with a 'patient information sheet' about the procedure itself, as well as further guidance on additional tests and investigations. Postoperative advice on discharge and any likely follow-up information was also included. Du Rand and colleagues (2013) have suggested how verbal and, in particular written, patient information can improve 'the tolerance of the procedure'. It may also help to alleviate patient fear and anxiety levels (Poi et al., 1998).

Given Spiros's symptoms and presenting history, and the likelihood of possible carcinoma, blood tests for platelet count and prothrombin time were requested in case a transbronchial biopsy was required. This is necessary to check for normal blood clotting and to prevent the likelihood of excessive bleeding. Although not appropriate to Spiros, patients on anticoagulant medication should be advised to stop taking their medication at least three days before the procedure. In Spiros's case, spirometry testing as a result of suspected chronic obstructive pulmonary disease (COPD) was not undertaken, and antibiotic prophylaxis due to previous diagnosis of endocarditis or prosthetic heart valve replacement was also not deemed necessary. On the day of the procedure Spiros was advised not to eat for four hours preoperatively but that he could have clear fluids by mouth (small sips) up to two hours before his bronchoscopy. Due to the effects of sedation Spiros was informed that he would not be allowed to drive and that he would need someone to accompany him home.

Stop and think

What the indications and adverse effects associated with bronchoscopy?

Indications for diagnostic bronchoscopy

- Persistent or unexplained cough
- Haemoptysis (blood in the sputum)
- Abnormal chest radiograph such as a mass, nodule or inflammation in the lung
- Removal of inhaled foreign body
- Evaluation of a possible lung infection
- Bronchial biopsy
- Bronchoalveolar lavage (BAL) to enable cell counts, cytology and culture

Severe adverse effects of bronchoscopy

- Severe bleeding
- Cardiac arrhythmia requiring treatment
- Seizures
- Myocardial infarction/pulmonary oedema
- Pneumothorax requiring aspiration/drainage
- Over-sedation requiring ventilation or reversal
- Hospitalisation
- Admission to intensive care unit
- Death

Source: Adapted from Du Rand *et al.* (2013)

5 **Consider and describe the preparation of the clinical environment and equipment needed to care for Spiros.**

A It is usually the case that bronchoscopy is carried out in a specific endoscopy suite, but on occasion it can be carried out in a range of clinical settings, including the operating theatre. Although endoscopy suites are normally staffed by nurses, the staffing level and skill mix is dictated by the number of procedures, availability of rooms, the ability to care for patients under sedation, as well as the adverse effects of sedative drugs, which require careful monitoring during and after the procedure. This skill set is in many ways similar to that of the ODP and a number of practitioners spend some of their time working specifically in endoscopy suites caring for patients undergoing flexible bronchoscopy. Many other ODPs may also be involved with bronchoscopy as a procedure carried out in the operating theatre, and this may include both flexible and rigid bronchoscopy.

Issues of legal and professional accountability that apply to ODPs carrying out the perioperative role have been clearly identified (Wordsworth, 2007) and, more recently, maintaining registration in advanced or extended scope of practice has also been discussed. Therefore it is imperative that ODPs who work in endoscopy/bronchoscopy are able to exercise their professional judgement and do not undertake activities for which they are not competent or in which they are not proficient (Wordsworth, 2014).

Infection control and prevention measures that apply to the physical space within the operating theatre also apply to the endoscopy suite. Preparation of the broncho-scope itself was undertaken by staff using appropriate personal protective equip-ment (PPE) (gloves, aprons, visors or goggles, face mask and forearms covered).

The bronchoscope itself is essentially a long, flexible fibre-optic hollow tube. At one end is a body that allows a light source and an optical lens or camera to be fitted. A control lever allows the tip of the bronchoscope to bend and flex to various angles to enable the instrument to be manipulated down into the bronchial tree. Various ports allow suction or ventilation to take place; these make it possible to pass instruments such as forceps through the scope in order to undertake biopsies, brushings or lavage.

After each use, a leak test and manual cleaning of the bronchoscope with water and detergent should take place. Suction and biopsy channels are cleaned with a single-use brush, and then irrigated with detergent, followed by water and finally air. The scope is then rinsed and placed in an automated endoscope reprocessor (AER) for further disinfection using the manufacturer's approved cleaning agent. The scope is then dried, and hung and stored appropriately ready for its next use.

6   **Evaluate key aspects of the care of the sedated patient undergoing bronchoscopy.**

 Spiros attended the endoscopy unit as a day case patient accompanied by his wife, and therefore did not receive a pre-medication. The bronchoscopist explained the procedure to Spiros in full, including the associated risks. She also talked through the need for sedation, and explained how he may feel while undergoing a bronchoscopy; some patients might find the sensation unsettling if not painful. At the end of this dialogue Spiros was able to provide his informed consent.

Once in the bronchoscopy suite Spiros was positioned in a sitting-up position (although the procedure can be performed with the patient supine) and venous access was secured in his non-dominant hand. Without the need for an anaesthetic, bronchoscopy is tolerated well using sedation to the level of 'conscious sedation' in accordance with the hospital's safe sedation policy (Table 11.1 assessment/ sedation scale). This meant that, throughout the procedure, Spiros was able to main-tain his own airway patency and cardio-respiratory function; he was also able to respond verbally throughout. According to the British Thoracic Society (BTS) good practice guidelines (Du Rand *et at.*, 2013), a 5 ml rather than a 10 ml syringe of low-strength midazolam (1 mg/ml) was prepared in readiness. Low strengths of the drug, as opposed to 2 mg or 5 mg/ml, or indeed propofol, which only has a short therapeutic window, allowed administration by the bronchoscopist rather than an anaesthetist.

Prior to insertion of the bronchoscope, 1% lidocaine was sprayed into the back of Spiros's throat. Topical anaesthesia again using 1% lidocaine but in gel form, was also administered nasally to aid the passage of the scope through the trans-nasal passages. Spiros was feeling very nervous before the procedure and had expressed some surprise in his own words that he would not be 'put to sleep'. Afterwards Spiros recalled the feeling of the scope as it was passed down through his nose as being

Table 11.1   Modified observer's assessment of alertness/sedation (MOAAS) scale

Level	Response
5	Responds readily to name spoken in normal tone
4	Lethargic response to name spoken in normal tone
3	Responds only after name is called loudly or repeatedly
2	Responds only after mild prodding or shaking
1	Does not respond to mild prodding or shaking
0	Does not respond to pain

Source: Chernik *et al.* (1990)

'really weird'. A 1% solution of lidocaine was administered through the working channel of the bronchoscope using a 'spray as you go' technique, to prevent irritation and reduce cough and stridor as the scope was passed through the vocal cords and on into the trachea. Spiros suggested afterwards that although this felt a little uncomfortable, the procedure was not painful. However, the spray tasted 'a bit like banana flavour', which he described as 'disgusting'. Worse still, Spiros felt that his throat was swelling up slightly, in addition to which the gel stung and this made his eyes water.

From the outset, during and after the procedure, Spiros's heart rate, blood pressure and oxygen saturation were monitored; the latter was particularly important as sedation and the passage of the scope through the vocal cords can lead to hypoxaemia, typically indicated in a fall of more than 4% SpO_2 or an SpO_2 of less than 90%.

7   **Describe the technique of bronchoscopy.**

A   Before the procedure commenced, an adaptation of the WHO safety checklist for bronchoscopy was carried out. Further checks were made immediately prior to sedation and then again at the end of the procedure. Once the bronchoscopist was ready she checked with Spiros that he was happy to continue; the tip of the bronchoscope was initially passed through Spiros's nasal cavity and guided through the pharynx and larynx to the vocal cords. Spiros was asked to make different sounds to check the range of movement of the vocal cords, which appeared completely normal; otherwise this may indicate invasion of a tumour to the mediastinum. The scope was then passed through the trachea to the carina, which was observed to be normal, before the scope was then inserted into the right main bronchus, thus inspecting each specific area as the scope was advanced.

The tip of the bronchoscope was guided carefully along the superior lobar bronchus towards the site identified in the CT scan. Careful examination followed of the junction of the anterior and posterior bronchiole, which again was normal. However, a small but well-defined smooth lesion situated on the mucosal lining was apparent at the junction between the posterior and apical bronchiole, typical of a carcinoid tumour. Observation in this way helped to accurately assess not only the exact location of the tumour but also staging according to the appearance of the tumour, involvement of nodes or likelihood of metastasis (TNM) (Mirsadraee *et al.*, 2012).

The bronchoscopist kept explaining to Spiros what was happening, particularly as she was preparing to take biopsies of the tumour and the surrounding tissue. With the lesion in clear view biopsy forceps were advanced in the closed position through the working port of the bronchoscope. Once at the distal end, an assistant helped to secure the bronchoscope from sudden movement, and the bronchoscopy nurse (under the guidance of the bronchoscopist) was responsible for deploying the forceps mechanism at the proximal end of the bronchoscopy. Clear visualisation was helped by fitting a camera system to the scope so that the procedure could be visualised via a high definition screen, yet slightly out of Spiros's view as he had expressed a wish to avoid seeing anything 'gory'.

In an open position and advanced to the target area, the forceps were closed to grasp as much tissue as possible. At this point the forceps were withdrawn up through the working channel of the bronchoscope. Spiros later recalled feeling an odd sensation of tugging, but without any pain whatsoever. NICE guidelines developed by Du Rand et al. (2013) recommend that five or six separate biopsies are taken from the lesion itself, as well as the surrounding tissue, in order to improve the diagnostic yield of tumour staging. Once biopsies had been completed, the bronchoscopist checked for any signs of obvious and abnormal bleeding, and felt that the administration of adrenaline 1/1000 diluted in 0.9% saline was not necessary, although it was readily available during the procedure.

Accurate gauging of the size and spread of the tumour is also improved by undertaking endobronchial brushings, which are necessary to gain an accurate cytological sample of the lesion and surrounding mucosa. Again the working port is used to enable the bronchial brush to pass through the bronchoscope until it can be viewed at the distal end. When the brush is pushed out it opens automatically from within a sheath, and is then advanced to the lesion and brushed over the surface several times. Once retracted into the sheath the bronchoscopist removed the brush up through the working port. In Spiros's case a further diagnostic procedure in the form of bronchoalveolar lavage (BAL), to identify disease or infection of the alveolar parenchyma was not carried out. With the specimens now taken, both biopsies and brushings were labelled carefully and checked against the patient's name according to the WHO (2008) Surgical Safety Checklist. At this point the bronchoscope was carefully removed and, because of the degree of conscious sedation, Spiros was able to discuss his experiences immediately after the procedure was concluded.

8   **What is the optimum post-sedation care of the patient up to discharge?**

A   Spiros was placed in a supine position and allowed to recover from the effects of sedation while his vital signs continued to be monitored for an hour after the procedure. Because Spiros's respiratory reserve was not reduced beforehand, supplemental oxygen was not administered during the procedure, although bronchoscopy can decrease oxygen saturation. However, as a precaution he was given supplemental oxygen after the procedure, at a rate of 2 litres per minute via a nasal catheter to ensure that his SpO_2 levels remained within normal limits. Throughout his recovery period, any changes in Spiros's respiratory pattern or onset of any chest pain should be closely observed, recorded and acted upon.

Gradually Spiros could feel the effects of the sedation wearing off; he felt less drowsy and more responsive to verbal commands. The strange taste and feelings in his throat had completely gone and he reported that he was not in any pain. With the effects of the local anaesthesia on his airway now gone, along with the return of his swallowing reflex, he was able to sit up and have a small drink of water.

Before being discharged Spiros's cannula was removed, and the bronchoscopist described the procedures that had been undertaken and her initial findings. Spiros's wife was there to collect him and both were given detailed discharge information that highlighted any specific complications they should be vigilant in looking out for (such as blooding and difficulty in breathing). Contact details of the bronchoscopy unit were provided and Spiros was encouraged to get in touch with them should he wish to. It was reiterated to Spiros that he should not drive or operate any machinery for at least 24 hours. He then left the unit with a written follow-up appointment.

Q **Discuss the follow-up and longer-term care of the patient.**

A At the follow-up appointment the diagnosis of a bronchial carcinoid tumour was confirmed. Spiros was informed that this type of malignancy is typically found in the segmental or larger bronchus, which is more common in men, and in which smoking is considered the most important causation. The positive news was that the tumour had been detected early and was classified according to TNM staging classification as T1A. This means that the tumour was less than 2 cm in length (in this case the tumour extended to a visible distal margin of 1 cm), with no evidence of nodal or metastatic involvement (Mirsadraee *et al.*, 2012). That said, only 5.5% of 39,000 newly diagnosed patients with lung cancer are cured (NICE, 2011).

It was recommended and discussed with Spiros that tumours of the type and nature he was diagnosed with are treated surgically, often involving segmentectomy or wedge resection to avoid the possibility of the disease reoccurring. Treatment options for so-called non-small cell lung cancer (NSCLC) can also include radical radiotherapy treatment. A combination of treatments, including radiotherapy and chemotherapy, is normally reserved for patients who are deemed to be not fit enough to undergo surgery (NICE, 2011).

Advanced bronchoscopic techniques also enable not only diagnostic interventions but are increasingly used to provide more therapeutic benefits, particularly in the form of electrocautery on early-stage malignant tumours with a visible distal margin and with invasion of the bronchial mucosa of less than 3 mm, as well as Nd:YAG (neodymium-doped yttrium aluminium garnet) laser to provide curative and de-bulking of tumours (Du Rand *et al.*, 2011).

REFERENCES AND FURTHER READING

British Thoracic Society (BTS) (2014) Bronchoscopy: patient information leaflet. Available online at: www.brit-thoracic.org.uk/…information/…/bts-patient-information (accessed 2 August 2014).
Cancer Care UK (2016) Lung cancer risks and causes. Available online at: www.cancerresearchuk.org/about-cancer/type/lung-cancer/about/lung-cancer-risks-and-causes#family (accessed 21 January 2016).

Chernik, D.A., Gillings, D., Laine, H., Hendíer, J., Silver, J.M., Davidson, A.B., Schwarm, E.M. and Seigel, J.L. (1990) Validity and reliability of the Observer's Assessment of Alertness/ Sedation Scale: study with intravenous midazolam. *Journal of Clinical Psychopharmacology*, **10**(4): 244–251.

Du Rand, I.A, Barber, P.V., Goldring, J., Lewis, R.A., Mandal, S., Munavvar, M., Rintoul, R.C., Shah, P.L., Singh, S., Slade, M.J. and Woolley, A. (2011) British Thoracic Society (BTS) guideline for advanced diagnostic and therapeutic flexible bronchoscopy in adults. British Thoracic Society Interventional Bronchoscopy Guideline Group. *Thorax: An International Journal of Respiratory Medicine*, **66**, November, Supplement 3.

Du Rand, I., Blaikley, A., Booton, J.R., Chaudhuri, N., Gupta, V., Khalid, S., Mandal, K., Martin, J., Mills, J., Navani, N., Rahman, N.M., Wrightson, J.M. and Munavvar, M. (2013) Guideline for diagnostic flexible bronchoscopy in adults. British Thoracic Society (BTS) Flexible Bronchoscopy Guideline Group. *Thorax: An International Journal of Respiratory Medicine*, **68**, August, Supplement 1.

Mirsadraee, S., Oswal, D., Alizadeh, Y., Caulo, A., van Beek, E. (2012) The 7th lung cancer TNM classification and staging system: review of the changes and implications. *World Journal of Radiography*, **4**(4): 128–134.

Morice, A.H., McGarvey, L. and Pavord, I. (2006) Recommendations for the management of cough in adults. British Thoracic Society Cough Guideline Group. *Thorax: An International Journal of Respiratory Medicine*, **61**, Supplement 1: 1–24.

National Institute for Heath and Clinical Excellence (NICE) (2011) Lung cancer: the diagnosis and treatment of lung cancer. *NICE Clinical Guideline 12*, April.

Poi, P.J., Chuah S.Y., Srinivas, P. and Liam, C.K. (1998) Common fears of patients undergoing bronchoscopy. *European Respiratory Journal*, **11**: 1147–1149.

Wordsworth, S. (2007) Accountability in perioperative practice, in Smith, B., Rawlings, P., Jones, C. and Wicker, P. (eds) *Core Topics in Operating Department Practice: Anaesthesia and Intensive Care*. Cambridge: Cambridge University Press.

Wordsworth, S. (2014) Professional practice and the operating department practitioner, in Abbott, H. and Booth, H. (eds) *Foundations in Operating Department Practice*. London: Open University Press.

World Health Organization (WHO) (2008) *WHO Surgical Safety Checklist and Implementation Manual*. World Alliance for Patient Safety. Available online at: www.who.int/patientsafety/ safesurgery/ss_checklist/en/ (accessed 20 January 2016).

CASE STUDY 12

Surgical fixation of fractured mandible: the care of Christopher Jones (CJ)

Katie Hide

INTRODUCTION AND LEARNING OUTCOMES

Fractures of the mandible are a common facial injury, and young men between the ages of 17 and 30 form the highest percentage of patients within this category. Interpersonal violence accounts for the majority of cases within this age group, with alcohol intoxication as a contributing factor. The male to female ratio has been quoted as being from 6:1 to 21:1, with the peak incidence at weekends and in the spring. Consensual evidence from studies conducted over the past decade (Lee 2008; Venugopal et al., 2009; van Hout et al., 2012; Rashid et al., 2013) states that the mandibular angle is one of the most common fracture sites resulting from interpersonal violence.

Patients presenting with mandibular fractures requiring fixation will undergo hospital admission and surgical intervention. Any presenting co-morbidities will impact on the holistic delivery of care throughout their perioperative journey.

By the end of this case study you will be able to:

- understand the sociological contributing factors to mandibular fracture
- discuss the principles underlying maxillofacial anaesthesia and surgery
- explain the importance of human factors for effective communication and patient safety
- provide a brief overview of sickle cell disease in perioperative care.

Case outline

Christopher Jones (who likes to be called CJ), a 23-year-old black male, is a Naval Rating who was enjoying weekend shore leave with friends. His Saturday-night celebrations ended early on the Sunday morning, however, following a violent altercation with two unknown males.

He arrived in the local hospital's emergency department (ED) via a Ministry of Defence police van, presenting with facial bruising and swelling, an abnormal appearance of the left lower jaw with associated minimal movement, including tenderness and pain, and some lower lip numbness. Movement of the lower left molars was also evidenced.

CJ is of mixed racial descent and, on joining the Royal Navy four years ago, routine health checks confirmed a positive result for sickle cell from his blood test. Sickle cell results from a mutation in the β-globin chain of haemoglobin (Hb), and further haematology tests showed that CJ had inherited one abnormal Hb gene, Hb-SA, making him a carrier and giving him a diagnosis of sickle cell heterozygous trait. Unlike sickle cell disease (SCD), which has two abnormal Hb genes (Hb-SS), CJ has less than 50% of abnormal Hb, resulting in a normal blood count and normal Hb levels (Purday, 2007). As a child (with an immature immune system) CJ was prescribed daily prophylactic penicillin to prevent the bacterial infections that cause increased sickling, resulting in acute exacerbations of painful 'vaso-occlusions' and 'acute chest' – two common crises of SCD. Other triggering agents of acute exacerbations include hypoxia, dehydration, acidosis, hypothermia and pain. Folic acid, essential for red and white blood cell production, was also prescribed daily for CJ and he currently maintains his 1 mg daily dose.

Stop and think

Find out more about sickle cell disease (SCD).

Populations that have SCD most commonly live in the 'malaria belt' around the world. Increased permeability of the sickle cell's plasma membrane causes potassium ions to leak out of the cell – this low cellular potassium level kills the malaria parasites infecting the cell. A person with one sickle cell gene therefore has a high resistance to malaria. Aggregation of the Hb in low-oxygen conditions results in sickling of the erythrocyte and the loss of cell elasticity: erythrocytes need to alter shape when travelling through narrow capillaries, returning to normal shape when oxygen tension increases. Sickle cells do not return to normal shape due to their decrease in elasticity, and this inability can result in occlusion of narrow vessels causing ischaemia and tissue infarction. The spleen destroys these misshapen sickle cells through haemolysis, but erythropoiesis in the bone marrow cannot match the erythrocyte destruction rate, and haemolytic anaemia results. Normal erythrocytes live for 90–120 days, but sickle cells live for only 10–20 days (Tortora and Grabowski, 2002).

Triaged as 'urgent' in ED (HSCIC, 1998) and assessed by the on-call maxillofacial registrar, CJ underwent plain x-rays and a computerised tomography (CT) scan that diagnosed a unilateral comminuted angle fracture of his left mandible. Although diagnostic ultrasonography for maxillofacial fractures has been deemed comparable to CT (Adeyemo and Akadiri, 2011), this tool is not yet in use in the local hospital. No basal skull fractures, sometimes evident with head/facial injuries, were noted. An open reduction and internal fixation (ORIF) were recommended to repair the fracture within the next 24 hours, and full discussion and consent would be obtained the next day.

1 **CJ was scheduled for surgery the following day. Why do you think this was? What care would he have required while waiting for surgery?**

A Repairing the fracture within 24 hours was determined as the most advantageous procedure considering CJ's age, fitness and Royal Naval career prospects. CJ was also anxious and kept stating that he 'just wanted to get back to the ship'. Alternative, closed treatment using arch bars with wires for mandibulomaxillary fixation (MMF) takes up to eight weeks to repair, whereas an ORIF has the advantage of direct anatomical realignment, early return to normal function, as per CJ's wishes, and minimal complications (AO Foundation, 2008).

CJ agreed to be admitted to the surgical ward, where, to prevent triggering of erythrocyte sickling, he was prescribed diclofenac sodium dispersible tablets, 50 mg eight hourly, a NSAID to relieve his pain, prophylactic erythromycin oral suspension, 500 mg six hourly, a macrolide antibiotic to prevent infection (BNF, 2015), and an intravenous crystalloid infusion of 500 ml isotonic Hartmann's solution, to maintain effective hydration in light of his reduced ability to take oral fluids. CJ's base vital signs were observed and documented, and were within normal parameters. Sleep, excretion of the alcohol, some reduction in facial swelling, and expert advice from a haematologist prior to surgery would all enable a safer surgical intervention for CJ.

2 **What preoperative discussions and preparation would the surgical team complete with CJ?**

A The maxillofacial consultant and the registrar met with CJ and they pointed out to him the fracture lines in the angle of his mandible, from the x-rays and CT scan. Information regarding the proposed surgical approach was discussed and the consultant answered all of CJ's questions (RCS, 2008). Informed consent for the ORIF was gained from CJ, with the planned surgery scheduled to take place during normal operating times, as research has shown a higher complication rate in maxillofacial trauma surgery during out-of-hours, compared with in-hours (Bertram, Hyam and Hapangama, 2013). The surgeon then marked the surgical site with an indelible marker pen and reassured CJ that the consultant anaesthetist and a haematologist would visit him that day to discuss his operative plan of care, including his sickle cell trait.

3 **What do you think the key components of CJ's anaesthetic assessment included?**

A The consultant anaesthetist visited and assessed CJ with regard to his anaesthetic and airway management (AAGBI, 2010; Watkins, Opie and Norman, 2011). Anaesthesia for maxillofacial surgery can be demanding (Chalmers and Elliott, 2011) as the airway is shared with the surgeon. The consultant anaesthetist soon gained a good rapport and working relationship with CJ, and discussed his medical history.

CJ had received no previous blood transfusions in relation to his sickle cell trait, had no known allergies, had not undergone any previous anaesthetics himself, but his English mother had – with no ill effects. The consultant anaesthetist was unable to utilise the airway Mallampati scoring system due to CJ's swelling and trismus, common features of traumatic mandibular fractures, and so indicated a definite 'difficult airway'. Physical examination as per AAGBI preoperative guidelines (2010) was within normal parameters, and CJ's health and fitness were commensurate with those of a member of the UK armed forces who is fit and well.

Information about and discussion of the different anaesthetic techniques available for the surgery found CJ dismissing regional anaesthesia with sedation in preference for a general anaesthetic as he said he 'did not want to be awake during it'. Regional anaesthesia consists of using a peripheral nerve stimulator to block the mandibular and maxillary nerves using 0.5% bupivacaine diluted in saline. Sedation is achieved with a titrated propofol IV infusion, with effective oxygen saturation maintained using a nasal catheter via a nasopharyngeal airway. Significant findings of regional anaesthesia suggest lower pain scores and reduced postoperative nausea and vomiting (PONV) (Rastogi *et al.*, 2014).

The consultant anaesthetist described the 'awake' fibre-optic nasotrachael intubation process to CJ, as conscious sedation was deemed the safest way to avoid the potential of hypoxia and acidosis on intubation, two of the triggering agents to erythrocyte sickling. All questions from CJ were answered and he verbally consented to this anaesthetic technique.

CJ consented to bloods being taken by the haematologist for full blood count and antibody screening plus 'group and save'. Discussion ensued regarding the possibility of a preoperative blood transfusion to increase CJ's oxygen transportation and reduce the number of sickle cells; however, as CJ had only sickle cell trait with normal blood counts, a blood transfusion was deemed not to be required. This decision was supported by the Cochrane Review by Hirst and Williamson (2010), who concluded that there is insufficient reliable evidence proving any benefit in SCD, and that in some cases transfusion associated circulatory overload (TACO) is a cause for findings of morbidity. The haematologist reassured CJ that he would monitor his blood regularly until he was fit for discharge.

4   **What additional preoperative preparation must be considered?**

A   CJ continued taking oral clear fluids until two hours prior to anaesthesia (RCN, 2005). He was also asked to self-administer one spray of the nasal decongestant, xylometazoline hydrochloride 0.1% (Otrivine) into each nostril to help reduce nasal mucosa and constrict the nasal blood vessels prior to nasotrachael intubation.

5   **How would you prepare the theatre environment for this case?**

A   All routine checks of the environment and working equipment were made prior to a team brief. The cleanliness of each area within the department was examined to ensure adherence to infection control regulations and standard precautions (Pratt *et al.*, 2007). The temperature in theatre was increased to 23°C to counter possible hypothermia to CJ – a sickling trigger agent (NICE, 2008).

6 **What aspects of CJ's care is it particularly important to discuss as part of the team brief?**

A The consultant anaesthetist informed the team of his anaesthetic plan and the conscious sedation fibre-optic intubation (Rodrigues *et al*., 2012) consented to by CJ, due to his difficult airway and sickle cell triggering factors. He asked that theatre staff could be readily available during the induction in case of unanticipated problems. He did not foresee any, however, as these had already been discussed with the anaesthetic ODP, and all possible necessary items of emergency airway equipment had been checked and were available.

The consultant maxillofacial surgeon informed the team that a submandibular surgical approach would be used as CJ had a complex comminuted fracture requiring greater access and manipulation than an intraoral approach could achieve (AO Foundation, 2008). His extra surgical requirements would include:

- small plates and screws for temporary MMF
- load-bearing fixation with locking 2.4 reconstruction plates and screws
- plate bender for individual contouring of the plate
- dental extraction set for removal of fractured second and impacted third molars, as these will impair the reduction and compromise the resulting fracture fixation.

The scrub ODP confirmed that all the required equipment for the osteosynthesis (fixation) had been checked and was available.

7 **What do you think is the best way for CJ to be transported to theatre?**

A CJ was collected from the ward by a member of the theatre team, who ensured that all necessary checks had been completed before walking with CJ to the operating theatre. Walking helps to optimise the respiratory and cardiovascular systems, thereby reducing the chances of postoperative chest/airway complications and venous thromboembolism (VTE), respectively. Walking also generates body heat, thus reducing the incidence of inadvertent perioperative hypothermia prior to anaesthetic induction and the intraoperative procedure (NICE, 2008).

8 **How would you prepare CJ for the induction of anaesthesia and support him during this process? You should also consider any equipment required and any pharmacological interventions.**

A The flexible fibre-optic scope was prepared with a size 7 mm nasal endotracheal tube (ETT) railroaded over it. Suction tubing was attached and working, and the light focused. CJ was welcomed by the consultant anaesthetist and introduced to the anaesthetic ODP on arrival in the anaesthetic room. He was made comfortable in a sitting position on a theatre trolley; routine monitoring of his vital signs commenced, and the WHO checklist 'sign in' (2009a) was undertaken and completed. CJ's aural temperature was recorded as 36.8°C – well above the minimum 36°C benchmark guideline for surgery (NICE, 2008).

Throughout the anaesthetic intubation, the anaesthetic ODP reassured CJ by informing and explaining beforehand every action performed by the anaesthetist, asking him to let her know if he felt uncomfortable at any time. This conforms to the healthcare ethical principles required in clinical practice, of autonomy, beneficence, non-maleficence and justice (Seedhouse, 2009).

CJ's existing IV cannula with Hartmann's infusion was examined using the Visual Infusion Phlebitis (VIP) scoring system; the site appeared healthy and the VIP score was 0. The anaesthetist administered 200 micrograms of glycopyrronium IV, an anti-muscarinic drug used to reduce salivary secretions. The nose was then anaesthetised using Xylocaine spray 10% into both nostrils. Supplemental oxygen 6 L/min was then administered continuously via a nasal catheter into the right nostril, and conscious sedation was achieved using a benzodiazepine, midazolam, 2 milligrams per minute and an opioid, fentanyl 0.50 micrograms per minute (Rodrigues *et al.*, 2012) titrated using an anaesthetic pump. The left nostril was anaesthetised with a nasopharyngeal (NP) airway lubricated with Instillagel (local anaesthetic) prior to insertion. Anaesthetising the mouth was problematic as CJ had only very limited mouth opening, but he managed with a straw to gargle and spit out some lignocaine 4% solution. Removing the NP airway, the flexible bronchoscope was passed through the nose and down to just above the vocal cords; 4 ml of lignocaine 4% was injected through the scope to anaesthetise the cords and, after a wait of one minute, the ETT was then railroaded through the cords into the correct position, and taped in to secure it in place.

Giving more reassurance and telling CJ he was now 'going off to sleep' the anaesthetist administered the general IV anaesthetic drugs: propofol for induction, reducing any 'hangover' effect and a more rapid recovery; fentanyl, an opioid analgesic, to enhance induction and reduce pain; and atracurium, a non-depolarising muscle relaxant with intermediate duration. Inhalational 3% sevoflurane, a volatile anaesthetic, with oxygen and nitrous oxide was administered for continued maintenance of anaesthesia (BNF, 2015) to ensure CJ was 'not aware' during the procedure. Prophylactic, macrolide antibiotic erythromycin was given IV, and with muscle relaxation the anaesthetist was able to insert a throat pack to protect CJ's laryngopharynx from soiling during surgery.

Ensuring that all monitoring cables and IV infusion lines were stable, CJ was transferred into theatre and positioned on the operating table using the recommended manual handling techniques and equipment. Using correct manual handling protects both patient and staff from physical injury. The anaesthetist connected the anaesthetic circuit to CJ's ETT and commenced intermittent positive pressure ventilation (IPPV) to maintain normocarbia reducing hypoxic acidosis crises, a trigger for erythrocyte sickling.

Q **How would you prepare CJ for surgery once he has been transferred to the operating table?**

A The anaesthetic ODP, having ensured the vital signs monitoring and IV lines were correctly connected, used gel pads and padding to protect CJ's pressure areas from pressure sores. A heating mattress was in situ on the operating table, to prevent CJ from developing hypothermia, in addition to a forced air warming blanket that would be put on after the anaesthetic ODP had applied a diathermy plate to CJ's right thigh. Some hair removal was necessary before the plate could be applied, to ensure good skin contact. CJ was supine on the operating table and, to protect against VTE, long leggings were put on his legs and attached to an intermittent pneumatic compression pump, which prevents venous stasis and the risk of deep vein thrombosis. When satisfied that CJ was safely positioned and anaesthesia was controlled, the surgical procedure began.

10 **Prior to the start of surgery what else must be undertaken to reduce the risk of errors?**

A CJ's x-rays and CT scan were displayed to prevent the 'never event' of 'wrong site surgery' and to show the theatre team the mandibular fracture. Before the start of surgery the WHO checklist 'time out' (2009a) was undertaken. All members of staff must attend, and no interruptions, talking or noise are allowed so that effective communication is maintained. Sterile instrument trolleys were brought in; the whiteboard was completed, documenting the throat pack in situ, and the number of swabs, sharps and other consumable items in use during the procedure (WHO, 2009b).

11 **What does CJ's surgery involve?**

A CJ was positioned in the reverse Trendelenburg position and a head ring put in place to steady his head prior to skin preparation and drapes being applied. A sterile field was established; this maintains asepsis and protects CJ from unwanted pathogens and microbes entering his surgical wound from 'unsterile' staff. The dental extraction of the 2nd and 3rd molars was completed and the surgeon then made a submandibular incision to access the fracture. Comminuted fractures have bone fragments that will not support the fracture and so require load-bearing fixation. The bone fragments were aligned and occlusion secured using temporary plates and screws to achieve MMF. The ORIF was completed using a 2.4 locking reconstruction plate with eight locking screws, four either side of the bone fragments. Locking plates and screws have advantages over conventional plates and screws as the plates do not need to have continuous contact with the bone, so do not compromise the blood supply; the screws do not loosen as they lock into the plate; this ensures no movement in the bone reduction. The reconstruction plate was shaped to CJ's mandible using a plate bender and secured to the bone with reduction forceps while the screws were inserted using a threaded drill guide that centred each screw into the plate holes. The temporary plates and screws for MMF were removed and occlusion rechecked before wound closure (AO Foundation, 2008). A suction drain was not necessary for CJ and the wound was closed in layers using absorbable Vicryl and skin closure with a clear 2.0 Prolene; Opsite spray completed the closure. Following the final count of swabs, sharps and instruments, and removal of the throat pack by the surgeon, the WHO checklist 'sign out' (2009a) was conducted. All documentation was completed, and oral fluids and a liquid diet prescribed.

12 **What do you need to consider when extubating CJ at the end of the procedure?**

A CJ's bed was brought into theatre and, when he was still lightly anaesthetised but able to maintain and protect his own airway against possible laryngospasm, the anaesthetist extubated him (AARC, 2007). An NP airway was inserted to enhance CJ's longer-term oxygenation as an oropharyngeal airway is contraindicated in patients with a gag reflex, trismus or oral trauma (Roberts, Whalley and Bleetman,

2005). CJ responded to voice and was transferred into his bed with the bedhead at a 45° angle. Oxygen was delivered via a Hudson mask at 6 litres per minute and he was transported to the post-anaesthetic care unit (PACU) accompanied by the anaesthetist and scrub practitioner.

13 **How would you assess and care for CJ in the post-anaesthetic care unit?**

A The PACU practitioner had checked all necessary equipment and, for continuity of CJ's care, was ready to receive him following handovers from the anaesthetist and scrub practitioner (AAGBI, 2013). The use of SBAR (Situation, Background, Assessment, Recommendations) from the NHS Institute of Innovation and Improvement (2004) assisted the communication of all relevant details regarding CJ's anaesthetic and surgical procedure. While attaching the vital signs monitoring, the PACU practitioner followed the standard assessment protocol (Hatfield and Tronson, 2009; AAGBI, 2013), as follows.

- AVPU is a neurological assessment using Guedel's four stages of anaesthesia and the returning reflexes. CJ was alert to voice and was at Guedel stage 1, with his bite, eyelash and eyelid reflexes all returned on arrival in PACU. He was verbally reassured as to his whereabouts in the PACU and informed that his surgery was 'all over'. Due to the action of anaesthetic drugs, hearing is the last sense to leave before anaesthesia induction and the first to return on emergence, so it was vital that CJ was reassured through listening to the PACU practitioner's calming voice.
- *Airway:* CJ's airway was assessed to ensure it was patent and that oxygen was entering the lungs with adequate ventilation. Without a clear and quiet airway, all other assessments are negated. CJ was sitting up and had a clear airway on admission, helped by the nasopharyngeal airway adjunct, and receiving 40% oxygen via face mask.
- *Breathing*: it is important to 'look, listen and feel'. CJ's respiratory rate was counted at 12 breaths per minute, and his chest was rising and falling equally on both sides. There were no wheezes, crackles or stridor heard, and his skin colour appeared to be perfused, evidencing a good level of gas exchange in his alveoli. This was confirmed by the pulse oximeter reading of 99% oxygen saturation.
- *Circulation:* CJ's radial pulse was felt, counted and recorded at 64 beats per minute. The PACU practitioner could also feel a warm, dry skin over the radial artery, indicating good perfusion and body temperature, plus a 'normal' pulse pressure indicating a satisfactory blood pressure (BP). These observations were confirmed through no evident cyanosis in the central or peripheral regions of lips, skin and nail beds; monitors read BP of 122/70 (mmHg) and aural temperature of 36.6°C. CJ's temperature was monitored, reducing the potential for hypothermia, another trigger for erythrocyte sickling.
- *Disability and exposure*: CJ had an uneventful emergence from anaesthesia, becoming more alert in a short time, possibly due to the fast reversal effects of sevoflurane. CJ's VIP score continued to be at 0, and another litre of Hartmann's solution was infused to ensure an adequate fluid balance. His wound looked healthy and was protected from pathogens by the Opsite dressing. Prophylactic anti-emetic IV ondansetron, a 5-HT$_3$ antagonist, was administered to combat

postoperative nausea and vomiting (PONV) as CJ's removed throat pack showed signs of moderate soiling, some of which may have drained into the oesophagus. CJ had also been administered IV morphine, an opiate that may cause vomiting, but as pain is a trigger for erythrocyte sickling, multimodal analgesics were required. Using the numerical pain tool, CJ assessed his pain as 3/10, 10 being the 'worst possible' and 0 'none'. Non-steroidal anti-inflammatory drugs (NSAIDs) were prescribed for CJ as rescue analgesia, but during his time in the PACU he remained comfortable and mainly pain free. Information giving, reassurance and maintaining CJ's dignity were respected throughout his time in the PACU.

PACU discharge criteria were achieved within 50 minutes and CJ was returned to his ward with NP airway in situ and oxygen at 4 L/minute – to be continued for 24 hours to reduce the potential for hypoxia, another trigger for erythrocyte sickling.

14 **What further care do you think CJ requires to ensure his continued recovery?**

A Postoperative x-rays were taken of CJ's osteosynthesis the next day for comparable study. He was managing to maintain an adequate oral fluid intake and his IV infusion was discontinued. He needed to maintain a healthy oral cleaning regime by cleaning teeth surfaces and gargling with chlorhexidine mouthwashes six hourly to prevent intraoral infection, a common complication following dental extractions. His antibiotics were continued for this reason when CJ returned to his naval base. He continued to follow a semi-liquid diet until he could manage firmer foods. Physiotherapy sessions with exercises for mouth opening began after hospital discharge, with the aim to achieve jaw opening of 40 mm within four weeks post-surgery (AO Foundation, 2008).

CJ attended an outpatient appointment one week post-surgery, where the surgeon checked the stability of his occlusion. A further follow-up appointment before his ship returned to sea was made for six weeks' time, when more check x-rays would be taken.

A follow-up appointment with the haematologist was also booked one week post-surgery and resulted in more blood tests for CJ. The results showed they were within his normal parameters.

REFERENCES AND FURTHER READING

Adeyemo, W.L. and Akadiri, O.A. (2011) A systematic review of the diagnostic role of ultrasonography in maxillofacial fractures. *International Journal of Oral and Maxillofacial Surgery*, **40**: 665–661.

American Association for Respiratory Care (AARC) (2007) Removal of the endotracheal tube – 2007 revision and update. *Respiratory Care*, **52**(1): 81–93. Available online at: rc.rcjournal.com/content/52/1/81.full.pdf+html?sid=402bd9cc-9053–478c-8f19–4551e08c8b6c (accessed 10 March 2014).

AO Foundation (2008) Mandible. Available online at: www2.aofoundation.org (accessed 7 March 2014).

Association of Anaesthetists of Great Britain and Ireland (AAGBI) (2010) Assessment and patient preparation. Available online at: www.aagbi.org/sites/default/files/preop2010.pdf (accessed 7 March 2014).

Association of Anaesthetists of Great Britain and Ireland (AAGBI) (2013) Immediate post-anaesthesia recovery. Available online at: www.aagbi.org/sites/default/files/immediate_post-anaesthesia_recovery_2013.pdf (accessed 10 March 2014).

Bertram, A., Hyam, D. and Hapangama, N. (2013) Out of hours maxillofacial trauma surgery: a risk factor for complications? *International Journal of Oral and Maxillofacial Surgery*, **42**: 214–217.

British National Formulary (BNF) (2015) *BNF 70*. London: BMJ Publishing Group Ltd/RPS Publishing.

Chalmers, A. and Elliott, S. (2011) What is new in maxillofacial anaesthesia? *British Journal of Oral and Maxillofacial Surgery*, **49**: 258–260.

Hatfield, A. and Tronson, M. (2009) *The Complete Recovery Room Book* (4th edn). Oxford: Oxford University Press.

Health and Social Care Information Centre (HSCIC) (1998) A&E initial assessment triage category. Available online at: www.datadictionary.nhs.uk/data_dictionary/attributes/a/a_and_e_initial_assessment_triage_category_de.asp?shownav=1 (accessed 10 March 2014).

Hirst, C. and Williamson, L. (2010) Preoperative blood transfusions for sickle cell disease. *Cochrane Review*. Available online at: www.thecochranelibrary.com/userfiles/ccoch/file/CD003149.pdf (accessed 10 March 2014).

Lee, K.H. (2008) Epidemiology of mandibular fractures in a tertiary trauma centre. *Emergency Medicine Journal*, **25**: 565–568.

National Institute for Health and Care Excellence (NICE) (2008) CG 65: Inadvertent perioperative hypothermia: the management of inadvertent perioperative hypothermia in adults. Available online at: publications.nice.org.uk/inadvertent-perioperative-hypothermia-cg65 (accessed 7 March 2014).

NHS Institute of Innovation and Improvement (2004) SBAR. Available online at: www.institute.nhs.uk/quality_and_service_improvement_tools/quality_and_service_improvement_tools/sbar_-_situation_-_background_-_assessment_-_recommendation.html (accessed 7 March 2014).

Pratt, R.J., Pellowe, C.M., Wilson, J.A., Loveday, H.P., Harper, P.J., Jones, S.R., McDougall, C. and Wilcox, M.H. (2007) National evidence-based guidelines for preventing healthcare-associated infections in NHS hospitals in England. *Journal of Hospital Infections*, **65**, February, Supplement 1: S1–64. Available online at: www.ncbi.nlm.nih.gov/pubmed/17307562_(accessed 10 March 2014).

Purday, J. (2007) Haematological disorders, in Allman, K.G. and Wilson, I.H. (2007) *Oxford Handbook of Anaesthesia*. Oxford: Oxford University Press.

Rashid, A., Eyeson, J., Haider, D., van Gijn, D. and Fan, K. (2013) Incidence and patterns of mandibular fractures during a 5-year period in a London teaching hospital. Available online at: www.bjoms.com/issues?issue_key=S0266–4356(13)X0009–9 (accessed 7 March 2014).

Rastogi, A., Gyanesh, P., Nisha, S., Agarwal, A., Mishra, P. and Kumar Tiwari, A. (2014) Comparison of general anaesthesia versus regional anaesthesia with sedation in selected maxillofacial surgery: a randomized control trial. *Journal of Cranio-Maxillo-Facial Surgery*, **42**: 250–254.

Roberts, K., Whalley, H. and Bleetman, A. (2005) The nasopharyngeal airway: dispelling myths and establishing the facts. *Emergency Medicine Journal*, **22**: 394–396. Available online at: emj.bmj.com/content/22/6/394.long (accessed 17 March 2014).

Rodrigues, A.J., Scordamaglio, P.R., Palomino, A.M., Quintino de Oliveira, E., Jacomelli, M. and Rossi Figueiredo, V. (2012) Difficult airway intubation with flexible bronchoscope. *Revista Brasileira de Anestesiologia*, **63**(4): 358–361.

Royal College of Nursing (RCN) (2005) Perioperative fasting in adults and children: 30. Available online at: www.rcn.org.uk/__data/assets/pdf_file/0009/78678/002800.pdf (accessed 17 March 2014).

Royal College of Surgeons (RCS) (2008) Good surgical practice. Section 4: 26. Available online at: www.rcseng.ac.uk/publications/docs/good-surgical-practice-1 (accessed 17 March 2014).

Seedhouse, D. (2009) *Ethics: The Heart of Health Care* (3rd edn). Chichester: John Wiley.

Tortora, G.J. and Grabowski, S.R. (2002) *Principles of Anatomy and Physiology* (10th edn). New York: John Wiley & Sons, Inc.

van Hout, W.M.M.T., Van Cann, E.M., Abbink, J.H. and Koole, R. (2012) An epidemiological study of maxillofacial fractures requiring surgical treatment at a tertiary trauma centre between 2005 and 2010. Available online at: www.bjoms.com/issues?issue_key=S0266–4356%2813%29X0005–1 (accessed 7 March 2014).

Venugopal, M.G., Sinha, R., Menon, P.S., Chattopadhyay, P.K. and Roy Chowdhury, S.K. (2010) Fractures in the maxillofacial region: a four year retrospective study. *Medical Journal Armed Forces India*, **66**(1): 14–17.

Watkins, T.A., Opie, N.J. and Norman, A. (2011) Airway choices in maxillofacial trauma. *Trends in Anaesthesia and Critical Care*, **1**: 179–190.

World Health Organization (WHO) (2009a) Surgical Safety Checklist. Available online at: www.who.int/patientsafety/safesurgery/tools_resources/SSSL_Checklist_finalJun08.pdf?ua=1 (accessed 10 March 2014).

World Health Organization (WHO) (2009b) Guidelines for safe surgery. Objective 7: 72–75. Available online at: whqlibdoc.who.int/publications/2009/9789241598552_eng.pdf (accessed 10 March 2014).

Total hip replacement: the care of Mary McKenzie

Claire Lewsey

INTRODUCTION AND LEARNING OUTCOMES

This case study examines the care of an elderly female undergoing elective total hip replacement surgery under regional anaesthetic. She suffers from osteoarthritis, which is a degenerative disease that affects the joints. The patient had undergone similar surgery to her left hip some five years previously.

By the end of this case study you will be able to:

- describe the preoperative care of a patient undergoing hip replacement surgery
- develop an understanding of all stages of a patient's perioperative journey while they undergo elective hip replacement surgery
- discuss some of the wider health and social factors that impact on elderly patients undergoing major surgery.

Case outline

Mary McKenzie is a 78-year-old female, who has a past medical history of chronic obstructive pulmonary disease (COPD) and osteoarthritis, affecting both her hip joints. Osteoarthritis is the most common type of arthritis in the UK and is characterised by the deterioration of the articular cartilage in synovial joints, particularly the knees and hips. The cartilage slowly roughens and becomes thin and damaged, while the bone underneath thickens. As it attempts to heal itself, the bone can become misshapen, leading to pain and reduction of movement (Arthritis Research UK, 2014). Mary has suffered from COPD for the past ten years, which in her case has been caused by chronic bronchitis. Having previously smoked 10–15 cigarettes a day, she was able to cease smoking following her diagnosis of COPD, which is now well controlled with a long-acting bronchodilator, which she self-administers via an inhaler with a spacer attached. She has an annual flu vaccination to reduce the likelihood of her developing chest infections.

Mary had a left total hip replacement five years ago, which has greatly reduced her left hip pain and improved her mobility. In the past year she has

---

been complaining of worsening pain and reduced movement in her right hip joint, which has not been adequately controlled with oral analgesia. This has left her unable to undertake her normal activities, such as shopping and housework, and this reduced activity has resulted in an increase in her body mass index (BMI) from 30 to 34. Following examination and x-ray, which showed joint space narrowing and large osteophytes, further surgery is now planned. The surgeon discussed the treatment options and possible complications with Mary and she was placed on the waiting list for a right total hip replacement.

1 **Given Mary's past medical history what preoperative interventions do you think were required?**

A While Mary was awaiting surgery she was referred to a dietician, who planned a weight-reducing diet for her. She found it hard to comply with the diet plan, but was determined to be successful as she realised that a reduction in weight would help both her present symptoms and her postoperative recovery. During the 12 weeks that she spent on the waiting list, her weight reduced by 6 kg to 92 kg and this resulted in her BMI falling to 32. As a BMI of greater than 30 is the standard classification for obesity, Mary was still categorised as obese and therefore remained at an increased risk of perioperative mortality and morbidity (Lotia and Bellamy, 2008).

Mary attended the pre-assessment clinic one week prior to surgery, where she had bloods taken for a full blood count and for urea and electrolytes, a chest x-ray and an electrocardiogram (ECG). The following baseline observations were recorded: pulse 82, blood pressure 140/91 mmHg, respiratory rate 16, peripheral temperature 36.2 degrees centigrade, peak expiratory flow 305 ml. As part of the Enhanced Recovery Programme, she was given comprehensive written information, which included pre-admission instructions and information about postoperative pain control, early mobilisation and the expected plan for her rehabilitation and discharge (NHS Institute of Innovation and Improvement, 2006). Due to Mary's history of COPD, and in order to assess her respiratory status, she was also reviewed by an anaesthetist. She established that Mary had had no recent exacerbations of her COPD and was not exhibiting any signs of active respiratory infection. She reviewed her chest x-ray and most recent exercise tolerance test, and concluded that her respiratory status required no further optimisation prior to surgery.

2 **Consider how the theatre environment was prepared in advance of Mary's surgery.**

A Routine checking and preparation of the anaesthetic machines, the anaesthetic room and the theatre equipment was undertaken. The use of unidirectional laminar flow ventilation has been shown to reduce infection rates in joint replacement surgery, therefore the vertical laminar flow system in the theatre was turned on prior to the preparation of any sterile equipment (Al-Benna, 2012). As Mrs McKenzie had multiple risk factors for developing inadvertent perioperative hypothermia, which included the length of her surgery and her American Society of Anaesthesiologists (ASA) grading of 3, a forced air warmer and a fluid warming device were also checked and prepared (NICE, 2008). Eschmann lateral brace supports and a Carter Braine arm support were collected in preparation for positioning Mary in the left lateral position. As this position is particularly unstable and requires multiple members of the perioperative team to support the patient during the positioning procedure, it was vital that the table attachments were easily accessible to facilitate prompt and safe positioning.

Prior to Mary being transferred to the anaesthetic room, a surgical brief was undertaken by the entire theatre team, at which the specific anaesthetic and surgical techniques were confirmed. The surgical practitioner noted the availability of the required instrumentation and of a full range of sizes of the prostheses that were to be used. The anaesthetic practitioner confirmed that a sample of the patient's blood had been grouped and saved in case a blood transfusion became necessary.

Stop and think

How would you optimise Mary's anaesthetic care?

Due to the existence of COPD, a spinal anaesthetic with a lumbar plexus block via a posterior approach was felt to be the safest anaesthetic technique for Mary to undergo, as it avoids many of the respiratory problems associated with general anaesthetic. She was anxious about 'being awake and hearing unpleasant sawing noises' and so as part of her care she was offered, and opted for, conscious sedation, in the form of intravenous midazolam, so that she was unaware of what was happening around her during the operation.

The anaesthetic practitioner initiated monitoring of heart rate (88), blood pressure (151/89), pulse oximetry (98%), respiratory rate (15), temperature (36.4°C) and ECG (sinus rhythm). These observations were recorded in the patient care plan, in order to have a baseline with which to compare future recordings. A size 16 intravenous (IV) cannula was inserted into one of the dorsal veins in Mary's non-dominant hand and an IV infusion of 500 ml Hartmann's solution was commenced. Hartmann's solution was prescribed in preference to 0.9% sodium chloride because balanced salt solutions, such as Hartmann's, are less likely to cause hyperchloraemic acidosis than 0.9% sodium chloride (Powell-Tuck et al., 2011).

---

3   **How would you have supported Mary during the spinal anaesthetic procedure?**

A   Mary was positioned in the left lateral position to enable optimum surgical access, the blood pressure cuff also had to be placed on the right arm and therefore, in order to prevent backflow of blood into the giving set during cuff inflation, a one-way valve was placed between the cannula and the giving set. To reduce Mary's level of anxiety, the anaesthetic practitioner then provided her with a clear description and explanation of the forthcoming procedures, particularly the importance of her cooperation during insertion of the spinal anaesthetic, i.e. in the sitting position with the spine flexed and the chin lowered to the sternum, in order to widen the interspinous spaces.

While being supported in the sitting position, Mary received a local anaesthetic infiltration to her skin using a strict aseptic technique. Lidocaine 1% was chosen for this purpose because of its rapid-onset. First, a 19 gauge introducer was inserted, followed by a 27 gauge Whitacre needle into the midline of Mary's spine at the level of lumbar 3/4.

Whitacre needles have a pencil point and are designed to separate, rather than cut, the dural fibres during insertion, and thus they aim to reduce the occurrence of post-dural puncture headache. The stillette of the Whitacre needle was then withdrawn, clear cerebrospinal fluid (CSF) was noted to flow from the needle, confirming the correct position and then, following aspiration of a small quantity of CSF, 3 ml of hyperbaric bupivacaine 0.5% was slowly injected. A hyperbaric solution was preferred because of its increased specific gravity, which results in the local anaesthetic tending to spread caudally when administered to a patient in the sitting position. The addition of an opioid to the local anaesthetic has been shown to prolong the duration of spinal blocks (Whiteside and Wildsmith, 2013), but, given the expected length of Mrs McKenzie's surgery, this was not considered necessary on this occasion.

Mary was asked to return to the supine position. She required assistance to do this as the sensation in her legs had become impaired due to the onset of the effects of the spinal anaesthetic. Her blood pressure was recorded and it was noted that it had fallen to 115/72 mmHg, which was likely to have been due to the sympathetic effects of the spinal anaesthetic causing vasodilatation below the level of the block.

4   **Describe the technique used to insert a lumbar plexus block.**

 After a few minutes, Mrs McKenzie was helped to turn on to her left side for administration of the lumbar plexus block. Immediately prior to insertion of the block, the anaesthetist and the anaesthetic practitioner confirmed the correct site by visualising the surgical arrow indicating site of surgery and by asking the patient to confirm the side of surgery, in line with the 'stop before you block' campaign (Safe Anaesthesia Liaison Group, 2011). The block was then inserted using peripheral nerve stimulation to aid placement of the needle. Mary was warned that she would feel muscle contraction in her quadriceps.

This technique relies on the anaesthetist and the anaesthetic practitioner working in unison. The anaesthetist inserts the insulated 100 mm needle, which is connected to a peripheral nerve stimulator and, once involuntary muscle contraction is visualised, the anaesthetic practitioner gradually reduces the electrical current until muscle contraction is no longer visible; the needle is then advanced further until muscle contraction reappears. The process is systematically repeated until muscle contraction can be stimulated with a current of 0.5 mA. If contractions are seen below this level, then there is the possibility that the needle tip is touching or has penetrated a nerve, so it must be confirmed that the contraction disappears when the current is reduced below 0.5 mA before any local anaesthetic is injected (Corner and Grant, 2013). Although not used in this case, ultrasound guidance is now preferred by some clinicians to aid the localisation of nerves, as other structures – such as blood vessels and muscle – can also be distinguished (Corner and Grant, 2013).

Once the needle position had been confirmed, a catheter was passed through the needle and secured in place, in order to provide a continuous lumbar plexus block for postoperative pain relief.

Stop and think

Which pharmacological interventions were essential to Mary's perioperative care?

The pharmacological interventions were as follows:

- hyperbaric bupivacaine 0.5%, 3 ml intrathecally
- bupivacaine 20 ml via the lumbar plexus block, intraoperatively
- bupivacaine 0.125%, 240 ml via a single-use elastomeric pump, which delivers 10 ml/hour into the lumbar plexus block catheter for postoperative analgesia
- metaraminol 10 mg diluted to 20 ml with sodium chloride 0.9% (0.5 mg/ml), for the treatment of hypotension from sympathetic blockage
- midazolam 1 mg/ml, for conscious sedation immediately prior to the commencement of surgery, titrated to effect
- tranexamic acid 1 g, to reduce bleeding, prior to commencement of surgery.

---

5   **Can you describe how the operating theatre was prepared prior to Mary's surgery?**

A   The scrub practitioner undertook surgical hand washing, gowning and double gloving, with inner indicator gloves, as this has been shown to aid the detection of glove punctures. The sterile instrument trolleys were prepared within the laminar flow, and the following specific hip replacement instrumentation was prepared and checked:

- basic orthopaedic instruments
- hip retractors (Charnley, and Norfolk and Norwich)
- battery-powered oscillating saw and drill
- acetabular reamers
- femoral preparation instruments
- trial acetabular and femoral prostheses, in a range of sizes
- acetabular and femoral prostheses insertion instruments
- cement restrictor sizing and insertion instruments
- bone cementing mixing system, with vacuum extraction and cement gun.

Once a full count of all the swabs, instruments and other accountable items had been completed, the instrument trolleys were covered with sterile drapes before Mrs McKenzie was transferred into theatre and on to the operating table. She was attached to non-invasive monitoring equipment, after which the entire theatre team paused to participate in a time-out procedure (WHO, 2008). Mrs McKenzie was then positioned in the left lateral position. Care was taken to ensure that her right arm was not over-extended, as this could cause pressure, stretching or compression of the nerves in the brachial plexus, which could lead to permanent nerve damage. Her head was supported by a pillow, to allow alignment with her cervical spine, and her left shoulder was brought slightly forward so that blood flow into her dependent arm was not impeded. Her position was secured with previously prepared table attachments and gel padding. The surgeon confirmed that the position was suitable before he began to scrub. Mary had only minimal hair growth in the area of the expected incision; hair removal was not deemed necessary, as this is not done routinely to reduce the risk of surgical site infection (NICE, 2013).

Following skin preparation with chlorhexidine–alcohol, which has been shown to be superior to cleaning with povidone–iodine (Lindsay, Bigsby and Bannister, 2011), Mary's right hip area was draped in such a way to allow manipulation of the joint during surgery.

6 **Can you describe a surgical approach frequently used to perform a total hip replacement?**

A A posterior approach was used, opening the hip joint via an incision on the posterior aspect of the greater trochanter. The joint was dislocated and the femoral head excised with an oscillating saw. The acetabulum was then reamed and prepared for the prosthesis. Following use of trial prostheses, the required size of press-fit (uncemented) acetabular shell and an acetabular insert were selected and checked by the scrub practitioner and the surgeon prior to opening. Before insertion of the acetabular shell, the scrub practitioner undertook a swab count to ensure that no swabs could be retained inadvertently beneath the prosthesis.

The proximal femur was then exposed, and the femoral canal was accessed and prepared using a box chisel, femoral reamers and then broaches of increasing size. Once the final broach was in place, femoral neck and head trial components were attached and a trial reduction of the joint was performed to confirm the appropriateness of the component sizes and their position. While the definitive femoral components were checked, opened and prepared for insertion, a pulse lavage and femoral brush were used to clean the femoral canal prior to the insertion of a cement restrictor.

Before mixing the bone cement – polymethyl methacrylate (PMMA) – another swab count was performed to ensure that no items had been retained in the femoral canal. The scrub practitioner then mixed the PMMA in a vacuumed mixing unit, to reduce its porosity (O'Dowd-Booth et al., 2011). The insertion of PMMA, particularly under pressure, has been associated with a number of adverse patient reactions, including transitory hypotension, cardiac arrest, pulmonary embolism and hypersensitivity reactions (Bowen, 2011). The reasons for these reactions are not fully understood, however a rise in intramedullary pressure causing the formation of micro-emboli and chemical/blood reactions have been suggested as possible causes. In the light of these known risks, the anaesthetist was informed when the bone cement was about to be inserted, in order that she could be extra vigilant in monitoring the patient's vital signs at this time.

Once the cement had reached the required consistency, it was inserted into the femoral canal and pressurised, before the femoral prosthesis was inserted and held in position until the cement had hardened. The circulating practitioner advised the surgical team of the time at 30-second intervals throughout the cement mixing and setting process. Following a trial reduction of the hip joint with a trial femoral head, a definitive femoral head was collected, checked and attached to the femoral component, before the joint was reduced and its range of motion checked.

7 How might Mary's wound have been closed?

A The scrub and circulating practitioners performed the swab, instrument and accountable items checking procedures in line with the local hospital policy, while the hip joint, muscle and subcutaneous layers were closed with Maxon and Polysorb respectively. Skin staples were used to close the skin. A literature review by Dignon and Arnett (2013) found that infection rates were comparable in hip and knee arthroplasty between using staples and sutures. They did highlight that skin staples have been shown to be quicker and easier to use, although they are more expensive than sutures. Therefore the evidence does not strongly favour one method over the other.

The wound was dressed with Aquacel, which was covered with a hydrocolloid dressing (Duoderm). Hydrocolloid dressings have been shown to help prevent superficial surgical site infection and blister formation in patients undergoing lower limb orthopaedic surgery (Siddique, Mirza and Housden, 2011).

8 Which aspects of Mary's post-anaesthetic care would you prioritise?

A On arrival in the post-anaesthetic care unit (PACU), the recovery practitioner was provided with a comprehensive handover, which included Mrs McKenzie's past medical history, details of the anaesthetic and surgical procedures, the blood loss (550 ml), her intraoperative cardiovascular status and her medicine prescription.

An initial assessment of Mary's postoperative condition was undertaken, which included assessment of her:

- airway and breathing – airway noted as being clear by using a 'look, listen and feel' approach, respiratory rate of 18 breaths per minute
- circulation – heart rate (81 beats per minute), blood pressure (132/85 mmHg), pulse oximetry (97% saturation), ECG (normal sinus rhythm), peripheral temperature 36.1°C
- level of consciousness – opened eyes to voice, assessed using Awake Pain Verbal Unresponsive (APVU) score
- pain score 0, using a 0–10 pain scale
- postoperative nausea and vomiting assessment – no nausea
- wound observation – no leakage visible through the dressing
- orientation to time and place – fully aware of place, required orientation to the precise time.

The level of spinal blockade was assessed using a covered ice pack, and initially Mary reported no sensation or motor activity at and below the level of her surgery. The lumbar plexus catheter and elastomeric pump were observed at 15-minute intervals for signs of dislodgement and obstruction. One hour after Mary arrived in the PACU she reported feeling 'pins and needles' in her legs and was able to make small movements with her feet. It was explained to her that this was a result of the effects of the spinal anaesthetic wearing off. At this point she reported her pain score as 2, and stated that she was not in need of additional analgesia.

Mrs McKenzie was encouraged to remain lying on her back with the abduction pillow between her legs. The colour, capillary refill, sensation and movement in both her feet were assessed. No leakage was observed from the wound dressing. Her oxygen therapy was discontinued 45 minutes after she entered the PACU; her observations continued to be monitored at 15-minute intervals, and were noted to be stable and within expected limits. After 90 minutes, Mary met the PACU discharge criteria and was transferred to the orthopaedic ward.

9 **What other therapeutic interventions were necessary to support Mary's post-operative recovery?**

A On the evening following surgery, Mrs McKenzie's observations remained stable, there was no leakage from her wound dressing and the continuous lumbar plexus block provided her with good pain relief (pain score of 2). The physiotherapist judged that Mrs McKenzie had sufficient motor function to be assisted to stand and she was able to stand with the aid of a Zimmer frame, despite initially feeling mildly dizzy. With the physiotherapist's assistance, she was then able to walk a few steps. The physiotherapist visited regularly over the next few days and, by Mrs McKenzie's fourth postoperative day, she was able to walk to the bathroom with the aid of crutches. She could also negotiate stairs, as long as someone was standing next to her. This was important because, although her house has a downstairs toilet, the bedroom and bathroom are upstairs. An occupational therapist assessed Mrs McKenzie and gave her advice on how to undertake daily activities, such as washing and dressing, and arranged for a raised toilet seat to be installed at her home.

10 **What holistic aspects of Mary's discharge from hospital would you identify as being important to her recovery?**

A Mary was discharged home on her sixth postoperative day, with written instructions about the exercises she must undertake and the measures she had to take to reduce the risk of dislocation of her hip. Her husband, who is elderly and frail but otherwise fit, was concerned that he would not be able to manage looking after his wife on his own, and so their daughter who lives nearby, moved into the house for a week. She was able to help with cooking, shopping, and particularly with encouraging her mother to undertake her exercises and to negotiate the stairs. After three months, Mrs McKenzie was able to walk unaided and had returned to all her previous social activities. She reported feeling rather tired, but also that she was pleased she had undergone the surgery.

REFERENCES AND FURTHER READING

Al-Benna, S. (2012) Infection control in operating theatres. *Journal of Perioperative Practice*, **22**(10): 318–322.

Arthritis Research UK (2014) What is osteoarthritis? Available online at: www. arthritisresearchuk.org/arthritis-information/conditions/osteoarthritis/what-is-osteoarthritis. aspx (accessed 12 September 2015).

Bowen B. (2011) Orthopedic surgery, in Rothrock J. (ed.) *Alexander's Care of the Patient in Surgery* (14th edn). St Louis, MO: Elsevier Mosby.

Corner, G. and Grant, C. (2013) Peripheral nerve location techniques, in McLeod, G., McCartney, C. and Wildsmith, J. (eds) *Principles and Practice of Regional Anaesthesia* (4th edn). Oxford: Oxford University Press.

Dignon, A. and Arnett, N. (2013) Which is the better method of wound closure in patients undergoing hip or knee replacement surgery: sutures or skin clips? *Journal of Perioperative Practice*, **23**(4): 72–76.

Lindsay, W., Bigsby, E. and Bannister, G. (2011) Prevention of infection in orthopaedic joint replacement. *Journal of Perioperative Practice*, **21**(6): 206–209.

Lotia, S. and Bellamy, M. (2008) Anaesthesia and morbid obesity. *Continuing Education in Anaesthesia, Critical Care and Pain*, **8**(5): 151–156.

National Institute for Clinical Excellence (NICE) (2008) CG65 Inadvertent perioperative hypothermia: the management of inadvertent perioperative hypothermia in adults. Available online at: http://publications.nice.org.uk/inadvertent-perioperative-hypothermia-cg65/guidance (accessed 12 September 2015).

National Institute for Health and Care Excellence (NICE) (2013) QS49 Surgical site infection. Available online at: http://publications.nice.org.uk/surgical-site-infection-qs49/quality-statement-1-personal-preparation-for-surgery#rationale (accessed 12 September 2013).

NHS Institute of Innovation and Improvement (2006) Delivering quality and value. Focus on: primary hip and knee replacement. Available online at: www.institute.nhs.uk/images/documents/Quality_and_value/Focus_On/latest_DVQ_path_Hip_and_KneePROOF_Nov.pdf (accessed 12 September 2015).

O'Dowd-Booth, C.J., White, J., Smitham, P., Khan, W. and Marsh, D.R. (2011) Bone cement: perioperative issues, orthopaedic applications and future developments. *Journal of Perioperative Practice*, **21**(9): 304–307.

Powell-Tuck, J., Gosling, P., Lobo, D.N., Allison, S.P., Carlson, G.L., Gore, M., Lewington, A.J., Pearse, R.M. and Mythen, M.G. (2011) *British Consensus Guidelines on Intravenous Fluid Therapy for Adult Surgical Patients*. Redditch: British Association for Parenteral and Enteral Nutrition.

Safe Anaesthesia Liaison Group (2011) 'Stop before you block' campaign. Available online at: www.rcoa.ac.uk/standards-of-clinical-practice/wrong-site-block (accessed 12 September 2015).

Siddique, K., Mirza, S. and Housden, P. (2011) Effectiveness of hydrocolloid dressing in post-operative hip and knee surgery: literature review and our experience. *Journal of Perioperative Practice*, **21**(8): 275–278.

Whiteside, J. and Wildsmith, T. (2013) Spinal anaesthesia, in McLeod, G., McCartney, C. and Wildsmith, J. (eds) *Principles and Practice of Regional Anaesthesia* (4th edn). Oxford: Oxford University Press: 124–135.

World Health Organization (WHO) (2008) *Implementation Manual: WHO Surgical Safety Checklist* (1st edn). *Safe Surgery Saves Lives*. Geneva: WHO.

PART 3
Suggested 3rd Year (Level 6) Case Studies

Abdominal aortic aneurysm: the care of George Grant

Mark Ranson

INTRODUCTION AND LEARNING OUTCOMES

Aneurysms were first described by early anatomists in the sixteenth century, who believed they were merely a widening of the blood vessel involved. While an aneurysm can occur in any blood vessel, aneurysms in the abdominal aorta are particularly common – accounting for approximately 80% of diagnosed aneurysms – and carry a high morbidity and mortality rate associated with the potential for dissection and/or rupture in large aneurysms, which is usually fatal. The precise pathophysiology of aneurysms remains unclear, however in a high proportion of cases they are associated with atherosclerosis, resulting in weakening of the elastin fibres that form the skeleton of the smooth muscle of the tunica media. The resulting weakening of the muscle wall causes changes in the shape and structure, which lead to enlargement of the wall as well as the lumen of the aorta. The widespread ischaemia, often associated with generalised atherosclerosis, potentially limits the function of major organs, resulting in co-morbidities such as coronary artery disease, which can complicate the care of patients with aneurysms. The most commonly accepted definition of an abdominal aortic aneurysm (AAA) is based on the diameter of the abdominal aorta, with an abdominal aorta diameter of 3 cm or more being considered aneurysmal (Wanhainen et al., 2008).

By the end of this case study you will be able to:

- explain the pathophysiology of aortic aneurysm
- discuss the preoperative preparation of a patient undergoing abdominal aortic aneurysm (AAA) repair
- discuss the anaesthetic care of a patient undergoing AAA repair
- describe the surgical care of a patient undergoing AAA repair
- discuss the post-anaesthetic care of a patient undergoing AAA repair
- discuss the long-term recovery prospects for patients undergoing AAA repair.

Case outline

George Grant is a 71-year-old male referred for assessment by his general practitioner (GP) for investigation and management of a one-month history of intermittent back pain. Initial investigation by George's GP led to a diagnosis of lumbosacral sprain, and management with bed rest and application of heat was recommended. However, this management plan did not improve George's condition and prompted the referral for further investigation.

Previous medical history

George has a 25-year history of hypertension managed with atenolol (beta-adrenergic receptor blocking agent). Twenty years ago, he suffered a myocardial infarction with subsequent follow-up and angiography revealing significant coronary artery disease. George underwent coronary artery bypass grafting (CABG) following his infarct, with good restoration of flow and supply to the myocardium post-procedure. Drug management post-CABG includes atorvastatin (a lipid-lowering agent) and aspirin (used here for its anti-platelet effect).

Presenting condition

George complained of back pain in the lumbosacral region radiating to the posterior aspect of his left leg. The pain was described as a dull achy sensation but was sharp at times. This has been occurring intermittently for the past four weeks with no previous similar episodes. The episodes of pain varied in duration, and George reported the severity of the pain between 5 and 7 out of 10 on a numerical pain rating scale. George had not experienced any lower limb weakness or tingling sensation, no weight loss or fever, and had not been involved in any recent heavy lifting. Walking was not interrupted by the pain, which appeared to be mainly aggravated by episodes of standing, sitting or driving.

Physical examination

On general observation, George appeared well nourished and well perfused. He was pain free at the time of examination and showed no signs of respiratory distress while sitting comfortably on the edge of the bed. Vital signs recording revealed a blood pressure of 145/85 mmHg, respiratory rate of 16 breaths per minute and pulse of 68 beats per minute, which was regular and of normal volume and character. His temperature was 37°C and oxygen saturation was recorded at 98% in room air. Examination of the lower back revealed no scars or deformities with no tenderness or warmth on palpation. A 50% limitation in lumbar flexion was evident but all other range of movement assessments were within normal limits. Lower limb neurological examination was unremarkable and revealed no deficits. Abdominal examination found a non-distended, soft and non-tender abdomen. No guarding or rigidity was evident on palpation of the abdomen, however palpation did reveal an expansile and pulsatile mass located predominantly above the umbilicus. No bruit (turbulent blood flow) was audible on auscultation, and bowel sounds were normal. Respiratory and cardiovascular examinations revealed no major abnormalities. The findings from this examination led to a differential diagnosis list, including abdominal aortic aneurysm (AAA), lumbar spinal stenosis, lumbar spinal strain, malignancy and degenerative origin (osteoarthritis). George was referred for further investigation.

Investigations

Blood tests taken at the initial assessment revealed normal urea, electrolytes, full blood count, erythrocyte sedimentation rate and C-reactive protein (CRP). An x-ray of the spine was performed and was normal except for visible calcification of the abdominal aortic wall. Abdominal ultrasound confirmed the diagnosis of an AAA with subsequent computed tomography (CT) scan showing an infra-renal AAA with anterior/posterior measurement of 6.5 cm and transverse measurement of 5.5 cm. Based on these findings, the decision was taken to electively repair George's AAA due to the high risk of dissection and rupture of aneurysms above a diameter of 3 cm. George was therefore referred for preoperative preparation for an abdominal aortic aneurysm repair.

Stop and think

Having read the case study, consider the physiology presented to you and the patient's past medical history. Can you see why AAA was included on the differential diagnosis list? If any of these terms or drugs were new to you, you may want to further your knowledge by reading about them.

1 **Prior to surgery, it was necessary for George to undergo a range of preoperative investigations; try to think of as many of these as you can based on the patient presentation provided.**

A George was referred to and reviewed by a vascular surgeon within two weeks of his initial diagnosis. The decision was taken, given George's medical history and presenting condition, to undertake an endovascular aneurysm repair (EVAR) given that this procedure has been demonstrated to carry an elective mortality rate of approximately one-third (1–2%) that of open repair procedures (Lederle et al., 2009). Given George's medical history of myocardial infarction and CABG surgery, and the high cardiac risk associated with AAA repair, an electrocardiograph (ECG) and echocardiograph were performed. While both of these investigations demonstrated evidence of George's previous cardiac history, there had been no deterioration in cardiac status or function since similar tests performed three years earlier. Due to George's cardiac history, he was already established on the medication regime recommended to optimise patient status prior to AAA repair. This included a beta-blocker for control of blood pressure, a statin for lipid-lowering effects and aspirin for its anti-platelet properties, therefore George's established medication regime was continued in the preoperative period.

A chest x-ray and arterial blood gas were performed to assess George's respiratory function and reserve, with these demonstrating no apparent abnormality. It is important to establish adequate renal function prior to undertaking AAA repair as blood flow and supply to the kidney can be affected by the aneurysm itself, the operative procedure being undertaken and the use of contrast medium for imaging during the procedure. However, in George's case the aneurysm was infra-renal (below the level of the kidneys) and the choice to undertake EVAR rather than an open repair procedure negates the need to cross-clamp the aorta perioperatively, thus minimising the risks of renal compromise during surgery. Renal function had been assessed at George's initial consultation and had proven normal. The images from George's CT scan were reassessed to thoroughly establish the size and extent of the aneurysm and its relation to renal vessels and iliac vessels due to the potential for compromised blood flow and supply to the lower limbs. Following preoperative assessment George was deemed suitable and scheduled for an elective EVAR.

2 **What do you need to consider when preparing the theatre for an EVAR procedure?**

A EVAR is achieved by inserting an endoscopic catheter into the aorta, usually via the femoral artery under radiographic guidance. For George's procedure, it is necessary to ensure that radiographic screening equipment is available within the theatre and the scheduling of the procedure needs to be coordinated with the radiography department to ensure that a radiographer experienced in perioperative radiographic screening is available for the duration of the procedure. Protection from ionising radiation is important, and it is necessary to place additional, mobile lead-shielding devices between the patient and theatre staff, as well as to ensure the availability of sufficient lead-lined aprons for theatre personnel who will need close contact with the patient during the procedure. As well as the availability of a suitable endoscopic catheter, other specialist equipment required for George's procedure includes the stent graft that is inserted through the endoscope to facilitate blood flow through the stent, thus isolating the sac of the aneurysm outside of the stent and minimising the risk of the aneurysm enlarging, leading to potential dissection and/or rupture. The facilities for conversion to an open procedure should this become necessary must also be readily available in case of complications during the endoscopic procedure; however, early studies have demonstrated that the incidence of conversion from EVAR to an open procedure is low at less than 1% (Smaka et al., 2011).

Stop and think

The location for performing EVAR procedures can be challenging as, while a conventional theatre is fully equipped for surgery and anaesthesia, accommodating the portable imaging equipment for endovascular surgery can be difficult. By contrast, many interventional radiology suites are not equipped for surgery. Consider the benefits and challenges of performing this procedure in each location, and the impact upon your practice and preoperative preparation. Then explore the literature relating to vascular hybrid operating theatres – do you think this offers a good solution?

3 **Considering George's past medical history, which anaesthetic technique do you think is most appropriate and why?**

A EVAR can be performed under either general or regional anaesthesia, although robust evidence of mortality and morbidity benefit of one technique over another is lacking (Smaka *et al.*, 2011). The anaesthetic options available were explained to George, together with the potential risks associated with each technique. In George's case, and with his informed consent, the risks of general anaesthesia associated with a co-morbidity of coronary heart disease led to the decision to perform his procedure under epidural anaesthesia. George was able to lie flat during the procedure, and the use of low-dose aspirin and its anti-platelet effects did not present a major risk for epidural insertion. One consideration that must be borne in mind when making anaesthetic choices is the prophylactic use of heparin as an anticoagulant during vascular procedures. While this does not prevent the use of epidural anaesthesia, the use of heparin during a procedure must be taken into account when planning for removal of the epidural catheter. The use of epidural anaesthesia also avoided the need for invasive airway management, with George able to self-ventilate with supplemental oxygen provided via a face mask to optimise oxygen supply and maintain arterial saturations above 95%.

4 **What monitoring would you prepare for George and why?**

A In addition to the minimum monitoring recommended by the Association of Anaesthetists of Great Britain and Ireland (AAGBI, 2007), an arterial line was placed in George's radial artery to facilitate accurate, beat-by-beat monitoring of blood pressure, thus allowing the prompt detection and management of any major rises or falls in blood pressure as the procedure was undertaken. Given the potential for significant blood loss if the procedure had to be converted to an open one, and the need to maintain good control over circulating fluid volume and blood pressure, a central venous pressure (CVP) line was inserted via the right subclavian vein to facilitate accurate monitoring of fluid volume status, thus informing fluid replacement management during the procedure. Due to the risk of renal impairment by the aneurysm itself, the operative procedure being undertaken and the use of contrast medium during the procedure, a urethral catheter was inserted to allow accurate monitoring of urinary output, aiming to maintain this at above 0.5 ml/kg/hour (Smaka *et al.*, 2011).

5 **How was George positioned for surgery?**

A George was placed in a supine position on a tilting, radiolucent table. Due to the loss of sensation and movement in the lower limbs resulting from epidural anaesthesia, pressure-relieving aids were positioned around George particularly at areas of bony prominence such as at the pelvis and ankle to prevent undue pressure on these areas during the immobility associated with the procedure. Intermittent pneumatic compression boots were applied to minimise the risk of deep vein thrombosis (DVT) formation during the operative procedure.

6 **How is the procedure performed and what must the surgical team consider?**

A The modern equipment used by the team in George's procedure facilitated full percutaneous access to the femoral arteries for insertion of the endoscopic catheter and associated equipment. It is, however, good practice to provide ready access to local anaesthetic such as 1% lidocaine in case of difficulty accessing the femoral arteries, necessitating a cut-down procedure to expose and facilitate access to the femoral arteries (Woodrow, 2011). Following insertion of the endoscopic catheter and progression to the site of the aneurysm under radiological guidance, aortic angiography was performed by the injection of a contrast medium via the catheter to confirm and establish the shape, size and position of the aneurysm prior to placement of the stent graft. The stent graft was placed with approximately 1 cm of length extending above and below the borders of the aneurysm to facilitate fusion with the healthy aorta on either side of the aneurysm and to prevent the potential complication of an endoleak (Robbins, 2010). These endoleaks are defined as a persistent blood flow outside the lumen of the endoluminal graft but within the aneurysm sac, and are due to incomplete sealing or exclusion of the aneurysm sac causing reflex blood flow into the sac. Following placement of the stent graft, angiography was performed again to assess the accuracy of the stent graft placement and to check for the presence of endoleaks. Following the successful insertion and positioning of the stent graft, the endoscopic catheter and associated equipment can be removed. In order to prevent haemorrhage and haematoma formation at the femoral artery puncture site, proximal (upstream) manual pressure was applied to George's femoral artery for ten minutes following the procedure (Smaka *et al.*, 2011).

7 **Consider the circulatory system. What specific monitoring and other considerations are required to maintain intraoperative homeostasis?**

A Blood loss during an infra-renal EVAR, as in George's case, is usually minimal, averaging approximately 200 ml, and the need for intraoperative transfusion is rare (Atwal and Wylie, 2014). However, prolonged procedures can result in ongoing blood loss from the access vessels, and complex EVARs can result in significant blood loss. The theatre team, therefore, were prepared with the availability of cell salvage equipment, a blood group and save was performed preoperatively, facilitating rapid access to blood should it be needed, and the provision of rapid infusion devices should blood loss be large and rapid. George's procedure was uncomplicated; his blood loss did not exceed the average of 200 ml and transfusion was not necessary.

The potential for ischaemia/reperfusion injury to the kidneys is eliminated in EVAR because of the brief and intermittent nature of aortic occlusion. Contrast-induced nephropathy, however, is an important concern. Due to the nature of the procedure, and the need for regular imaging to guide catheter insertion and graft placement, a significant dye load may be administered during angiography. With this in mind, during the digital subtraction angiography sections of the procedure George was asked to hold his breath as angiography was performed, thus minimising movement and the need for repeated contrast studies. Maintaining adequate hydration is also essential to ensure the maintenance of blood pressure and consistent blood flow to the kidneys. The insertion of a CVP line in George's case allowed constant monitoring of the venous pressure close to the right atrium, and while it does not measure blood volume directly it gives a good approximation of right atrial pressure generated by venous return to the right side of the heart. Using the transduced method of recording gave a continuous, monitored waveform and numerical estimation of George's CVP, and these readings were used to guide fluid replacement therapy with the aim of maintaining a CVP between 4 and 6 mmHg. Insufficient evidence exists on the benefits of any particular individual or combination fluid therapies (Toomtong and Suksompong, 2010) and, in George's case, while fluid requirements were relatively low, replacement needs were met by infusing crystalloid solutions to maintain CVP between the desired levels.

8 **While this EVAR is a minimally invasive procedure, it is still particularly important to monitor George's temperature. Why do you think this is?**

A Perioperative hypothermia is associated with myocardial ischaemia and arrhythmias. Given George's previous history of cardiac disease, this was an important consideration in maintaining intraoperative homeostasis. While the non-invasive nature of EVAR reduces the potential for heat loss during surgery, the theatre team were aware of this important consideration and facilities were made available to monitor George's temperature both prior to commencing the procedure and at intervals throughout, in line with (then) National Institute for Clinical Excellence (NICE) guideline CG65 (NICE, 2008). While George's temperature remained stable throughout the procedure, the need to increase the ambient temperature and the availability of forced air warming devices and fluid warmers allowed the team to be prepared to provide a prompt response to a fall in George's temperature, thus avoiding the potential complications associated with perioperative hypothermia.

9 **What would your priorities be for caring for George postoperatively in the high dependency unit?**

A Due to George's cardiac medical history and the potential for cardiac complications following surgical procedures on the abdominal aorta, the decision was made to transfer George to the high dependency unit (HDU) for initial postoperative care rather than transferring him back to the ward following a period of recovery. This allowed invasive arterial blood pressure and CVP monitoring to continue, thus facilitating the prompt detection and management of complications should they arise. Given the potential for cardiac ischaemia following the procedure, management in the HDU also allowed George to benefit from continuous cardiac monitoring for the prompt detection and management of potential cardiac arrhythmias. In addition to regular vital signs monitoring, George's epidural was also able to remain in situ to facilitate pain control during the immediate post-anaesthetic period and avoiding the need for early removal of the epidural catheter following anticoagulation therapy in theatre (the catheter ideally should not be removed for 24 hours to allow the anticoagulant effect to subside). Throughout this period staff were able to monitor the effectiveness of George's pain control while also monitoring his level of consciousness, respiratory effort, sensation and motor contol for potential complications associated with epidural pain control. Fluid management continued to be informed by continuous monitoring of CVP thus allowing staff to tailor George's fluid regime to maintain a CVP of between 4 and 6 mmHg.

Endoleak, as discussed earlier, is a potential complication of EVAR and if present will result in perfusion failure beyond the graft. With this in mind, and to allow prompt detection of any potential endoleak, George's pedal pulses were assessed on admission to HDU, marked for ease of location and reassessed initially on an hourly basis, as well as observing the general perfusion and colour of his lower limbs (Moll *et al.*, 2011). Careful observation of the percutaneous femoral access sites was also undertaken to monitor for any excessive blood loss or haematoma formation. Hourly urine measurements allowed staff to ensure that George's urinary output remained at or above 0.5 mg/kg/hr, to allow the prompt detection of and intervention to deal with any signs of renal impairment. George's immediate post-anaesthetic period was uneventful and he was able to return to usual ward care after 24 hours.

10 **Consider George's discharge from hospital. What ongoing care or monitoring do you think he may require?**

A Overall, George coped well with his procedure and felt relieved that this potentially life-threatening condition had been identified and managed promptly. He was discharged home on the fourth postoperative day with a follow-up home visit planned on the fifth day by the community healthcare team. George's previous infarct and CABG surgery had led to him acting on the advice of healthcare staff around a healthy lifestyle, and this advice was reiterated at his discharge following this procedure. Arrangements were made for George to undergo a CT scan on day 30 of his postoperative period, to assess for endoleak and/or graft migration. This proved unremarkable and George managed to return to his previous lifestyle with no adverse effects from the procedure. He was, therefore, put on to a schedule of yearly reviews, with instructions on the action to take should he experience a return of symptoms.

REFERENCES AND FURTHER READING

Association of Anaesthetists of Great Britain and Ireland (AAGBI) (2007) *Recommendations for Standards of Monitoring during Anaesthesia and Recovery*. London: Association of Anaesthetists of Great Britain and Ireland.

Atwal, G. and Wylie, S. (2014) Anaesthesia for endovascular aortic aneurysm repair (EVAR): anaesthesia tutorial of the week. Available online at: www.totw.anaesthesiologists.org (accessed 10 August 2014).

Lederle, F.A., Freischlag, J.A., Kyriakides, T.C., Padberg, F.T., Matsumura, J.S. and Kohler, T.R. (2009) Outcomes following endovascular vs open repair of abdominal aortic aneurysm: a randomised trial. *Journal of the American Medical Association*, **302**: 1535–1542.

Moll, F.L., Powell, J.T., Fraedrich, G., Verzini, F., Haulon, S., Waltham, M., van Herwaarden, J.A., Holt, P.J.E., van Keulen, J.W., Rantner, B., Schlosser, F.J.V., Setacci, F. and Ricco, J.B. (2011) Management of abdominal aortic aneurysms: clinical practice guidelines of the European Society for Vascular Surgery. *European Journal of Vascular and Endovascular Surgery*, **41**: S1–S58.

National Institute for Clinical Excellence (NICE) (2008) Inadvertent perioperative hypothermia: the management of inadvertent perioperative hypothermia in adults. *NICE Clinical Guideline 65*. London: NICE.

Robbins, D.A. (2010) Current modalities for abdominal aortic aneurysm repair: implications for nurses. *Journal of Vascular Nursing*, **28**(4): 136–146.

Smaka, T.J., Cobas, M., Velazquez, C. and Lubarsky, D. (2011) Perioperative management of endovascular abdominal aortic aneurysm repair. *Journal of Cardiothoracic and Vascular Anaesthesia*, **25**(1): 166–175.

Toomtong, P. and Suksompong, S. (2010) Intravenous fluids for abdominal aortic surgery. *Cochrane Database Systematic Review*, CD000991.

Wanhainen, A., Thermudo, R., Ahlstrom, H., Lind, L. and Johansson, L. (2008) Thoracic and abdominal aortic dimensions in 70-year-old men and women: a population based whole-body MRI study. *Journal of Vascular Surgery*, **47**: 504–512.

Woodrow, P. (2011) Abdominal aortic aneurysms: clinical features, treatment and care. *Nursing Standard*, **25**(50): 50–57.

Hemicolectomy: the care of Malcolm Edwards

Mark Owen

INTRODUCTION AND LEARNING OUTCOMES

The case study will focus on the unique care provided to a patient who has been diagnosed with colorectal cancer. The care provided from the initial appointment with the general practitioner (GP) through to discharge and long-term recovery will be considered. Specific focus will be placed on the surgical care provided, incorporating an enhanced recovery programme (ERP) protocol to improve the postoperative outcomes for the patient.

By the end of this case study you will be able to:

- explain the holistic care requirements for a patient diagnosed with colorectal cancer
- discuss the application of an ERP protocol to colorectal cancer
- identify the preoperative preparation of a patient for surgery
- explore the unique aspects of perioperative care for a specific patient
- analyse the case, and access further resources to enhance your knowledge and understanding.

Case outline

Malcolm Edwards is a 58-year-old male who made an appointment with his GP following symptoms of looser stools over a five-week period; he was aware that this may be indicative of bowel cancer (Cancer Research UK, 2014a). During the consultation Malcolm had a rectal examination with no swelling or lumps identified, with no lumps felt during application of pressure on the abdomen. The GP referred Malcolm for a colonoscopy and obtained blood samples for further testing, including anaemia and liver and kidney function (Cancer Research, 2014b). During the consultation the GP determined Malcolm's general health and his previous medical history including an occupational cause of mild chronic obstructive pulmonary disease (CODP) managed with a short-acting bronchodilator inhaler. Malcolm's initial patient information was recorded and is detailed in the accompanying box.

Initial patient information

Name: Malcolm Edwards
Age: 58
Height: 5 ft 10 in
Weight: 14 stone
BMI: 28.1 – overweight (30 would be obese)
Allergies: nil known
Mild COPD; non-smoker – no previous history of smoking
Alcohol consumption: 16–20 units per week
Occupation: independent farmer
Marital status: married for 38 years with three children – two daughters and a son (aged 36, 34 and 30, respectively).

Malcolm had tests for bowel cancer and the colonoscopy confirmed that there was a tumour in the ascending colon. The results of these earlier tests help to determine the staging of the bowel cancer. The TNM system indicates T for tumour (size of primary tumour), N for nodes (whether any lymph nodes contain cancerous cells) and M for metastases (whether the cancer has spread to other areas of the body). Alternatively, the Dukes' system could also have been used (Cancer Research UK, 2014b). Malcolm's staging was recorded as a stage 2 tumour, which has grown into the muscular lining of the colon, although the determination of lymph involvement is often confirmed postoperatively with pathological investigations. Biopsies taken during the colonoscopy will assist the pathologist in determining the grading of the cancer cells. The results of the biopsies indicated that Malcolm had grade 2 bowel cancer meaning that the cancer cells were moderately abnormal (Cancer Research UK, 2014b). The treatment option for Malcolm was to have a bowel resection to remove the cancer cells and removal of the associated lymph nodes in case cancer cells had travelled there too (Cancer Research UK, 2014b). Malcolm was scheduled for an open right hemicolectomy +/- ileostomy formation.

1 **What preoperative preparation do you think is necessary to optimise Malcolm prior to his admission to hospital?**

A Malcolm received a follow-up appointment with the hospital and this confirmed his diagnosis of bowel cancer. It is important at this stage to ensure that his fears and anxieties are reduced. This can be achieved by providing details of support organisations, leaflets and counselling, and encouraging Malcolm to discuss his feelings with a family member (Cancer Research, 2014b).

Malcolm had been identified for inclusion in an enhanced recovery programme (ERP) and, at this stage of the ERP, his GP arranged a follow-up appointment to ensure that Malcolm was optimised for surgery. With a BMI of 28.1 Malcolm was overweight and the GP recommended a weight loss programme including daily exercise; he also recommended that Malcolm consumed no alcohol for four weeks prior to surgery as this improves organ function and reduces postoperative morbidity and enhances recovery (Gustafsson *et al.*, 2013). The GP may also review the following as part of an ERP: test results for anaemia, diabetes and hypertension, and appropriate treatment as required (Enhanced Recovery Partnership Programme (ERPP), 2010). An assessment of Malcolm's nutritional status prior to surgery was completed by his GP and, as there was no indication of malnutrition, Malcolm was advised to eat normally prior to surgery with a minimal period of 'nil by mouth' (ERPP, 2010). An appointment was made with the colorectal surgeon in an out-patients clinic to discuss the surgery, associated risks and possible complications (Cancer Research UK, 2014b) to ensure that Malcolm was fully informed and involved in the decision-making process (ERPP, 2010). He was provided with the date of surgery during the consultation, and a preoperative assessment and preparation for surgery appointment made.

Stop and think

Find out more about the enhanced recovery programme.

An ERP is an evidence-based approach to providing patient care focused on a set of interventions that allow patients to recover from surgery with a reduced length of hospital stay and a faster recovery (ERPP, 2010; Gustafsson *et al.*, 2013). Three key areas are considered as part of an ERP: getting the patient in the best possible condition for surgery; best possible management during the perioperative phase of care; and best possible postoperative rehabilitation (ERPP, 2010). It is important to involve the patient in all stages of the pro-gramme and incorporate a multidisciplinary approach to providing an ERP. Specific tools have been developed for colorectal cancer within an ERP pro-gramme (Gustafsson *et al.*, 2013) and these will be incorporated throughout the case study.

---

2 **What preoperative assessments do you think would be undertaken?**

A As a patient on an ERP pathway Malcolm met specialist nurses who assessed his general health and provided specific information related to his surgical procedure. The consultation also provided an opportunity for the specialist nurses to explain the anaesthetic and pain management options, and allowed Malcolm to have his ques-tions answered (White and Rivett, 2012). The staff explained to Malcolm that it is not routine to see the surgeon or anaesthetist during the preoperative assessment, but he was provided with a contact number for the specialist nurse if he had any concerns regarding the surgery, and informed that an anaesthetic plan would be discussed and agreed with the anaesthetist on the day of surgery (White and Rivett, 2012). Risk assessments for venous thromboembolism (VTE) are routinely performed at this stage (Association for Perioperative Practice (AfPP), 2011) and Malcolm had his legs measured for anti-embolism stockings to ensure that the correct size was provided.

3 **What information do you think Malcolm needs to be given in the preoperative period to help him prepare for surgery?**

A The specialist nurses discussed the expected length of stay and the planned discharge date, providing Malcolm with an expected date for going home (ERPP, 2010). During the discussion Malcolm confirmed that he had arranged support from his wife and children following discharge, and that his son would be looking after the farm during his recovery (White and Rivett, 2012). As the surgical procedure includes the possibility of a stoma, Malcolm met with the stoma nurse to discuss the appliances and how to manage them (White and Rivett, 2012).

4 **What will happen when Malcolm is admitted for surgery?**

A Malcolm chose to attend the admissions unit on the day of surgery following a night at home in his own bed rather than staying overnight on the ward (White and Rivett, 2012). The admissions team advised him that he was first on the list and provided him with a gown and anti-embolism stockings. Malcolm met with the surgeon and signed the consent form for the procedure outlined above, including the associated risks and complications of surgery. Malcolm also met with the consultant anaesthetist, who took a brief medical history, and routine observations were recorded on the anaesthetic chart. These provide a baseline for further assessment, particularly during the immediate postoperative period (AfPP, 2011). The anaesthetist discussed the anaesthetic plan and explained the benefits of an epidural for postoperative pain relief as well as a reduction in the risk of postoperative nausea and vomiting (PONV), leading to a faster recovery. Malcolm agreed that he would receive a general anaesthetic with epidural for analgesia (Gustafsson *et al.*, 2013).

5 **What are the points for discussion at the preoperative team brief?**

A Prior to surgery a team brief took place (National Patient Safety Agency (NPSA), 2010; AfPP, 2011), which provided an opportunity for improved communication between team members and the open discussion of any patient safety concerns (NPSA, 2010; AfPP, 2011). This was followed by a review of the operating list and discussion of the equipment required, including sterile instruments, hypothermia prevention and VTE prophylaxis. The surgeon confirmed that linear staplers would be needed alongside a laparotomy set (other names may be used, but the essential instrumentation required is to enable the surgeon to access deeper into the peritoneal cavity, and use crushing and non-crushing bowel clamps as required). The surgeon also confirmed that there were no known allergies for Malcolm and no infection control alerts. The surgeon requested that intravenous (IV) antibiotics be administered in the anaesthetic room in accordance with the ERP, a minimum of 30 minutes prior to 'knife to skin' (ERPP, 2010; Gustafsson *et al.*, 2013).

6 **What needs to be considered when receiving Malcolm into the operating theatre?**

A Following the team brief Malcolm was sent for and walked to theatre (White and Rivett, 2012). During this time the anaesthetic practitioner prepared for the arrival of the patient. Essential preparations included checking the anaesthetic machines, preparing a size 9.0 mm endotracheal tube (ETT) and ensuring a sterile epidural pack was available, alongside syringe drivers. The anaesthetic practitioner took responsibility for checking in Malcolm and greeted him on arrival. Sign-in checks for surgery were performed (NPSA, 2010), and included identification of the patient, consent and skin marking. Malcolm had two identity bracelets on (AfPP, 2011) to reduce the risk of misidentification. The anaesthetic practitioner asked Malcolm to confirm his full name and date of birth, as well as the proposed procedure, and cross-checked these with the ID bracelets and consent form, and verified Malcolm's signature. Informed consent was valid in that Malcolm signed the consent form voluntarily and had the capacity to understand the intervention, including associated risks (Department of Health (DH), 2009). Malcolm was marked on the right side for the possible site of a stoma and this was checked by the anaesthetic practitioner (NPSA, 2010; AfPP, 2011). As part of his ERP Malcolm was permitted to drink water up to two hours prior to surgery and to take solids up to six hours prior to surgery (Gustafsson et al., 2013) this was confirmed with Malcolm during the sign in.

7   **What do you think the anaesthetic care for Malcolm involves?**

A   As part of Malcolm's ERP a standard anaesthetic protocol was required (Gustafsson et al., 2013) including interventions that reduce the risk of delays in recovery. Pre-medication sedatives were not prescribed as these have been shown to reduce post-operative mobility and affect oral intake of food and drink leading to a delayed recovery. During the intraoperative phase goal-directed fluid therapy was used as it has been shown to reduce both postoperative complications and length of stay in hospital (Allman and Wilson, 2011). The risks associated with PONV are factored into the choice of anaesthesia, including a thoracic epidural to reduce the requirements for long-acting opioids and a total intravenous anaesthesia (TIVA) with a remifentanil infusion (Gustafsson et al., 2013), which are short acting, allow a rapid awakening from anaesthesia and reduce the risk of PONV. Administration of 80% oxygen was also prescribed to help overcome the risk of PONV (Allman and Wilson, 2011), as well as simple analgesics for postoperative management of pain, including paracetamol and ibuprofen, reducing the requirements for opiates (ERPP, 2010). A number of receptors are involved in the development of PONV, therefore prescribing drugs that act on these different receptors as part of a multimodal approach to anti-emetics was employed, including ondansetron and dexamethasone (Allman and Wilson, 2011).

Once all essential checks were performed, large bore IV access was established and Malcolm was positioned for a thoracic epidural anaesthesia (TEA). The epidural catheter was positioned between T10–T11 thoracic vertebrae and a test dose of 3 ml 0.5% bupivacaine administered (Allman and Wilson, 2011). Malcolm was returned to a supine position and prepared for the administration of TIVA with a muscle relaxant to enable intubation. The neuromuscular blockade not only allows for relaxation of the vocal cords to enable intubation, it is also required to improve surgical access (Gustafsson et al., 2013). Intermittent positive pressure ventilation (IPPV) is used as a result of the neuromuscular blockade of the accessory muscles of respiration. A rapid sequence induction (RSI) was not performed as Malcolm was at low risk for aspiration. Laryngoscopy was performed and the ETT successfully placed through the vocal cords into the trachea, confirmed by capnography indicating expired CO_2, and auscultation of the chest for normal breath sounds and absence of sounds over the stomach (Allman and Wilson, 2011). As a result of Malcolm's earlier health assessment invasive monitoring was not indicated. As part of his ERP a nasogastric tube was not inserted, to reduce the risk of a chest infection and ileus following surgery causing a delay in his recovery (ERPP, 2010). VTE prophylaxis was achieved by the use of anti-embolism stockings and intermittent compression devices, while postoperatively consideration for early mobilisation with pharmacological prophylaxis for 28 days with low molecular weight heparin was prescribed (Gustafsson *et al.*, 2013).

8 **How would you position Malcolm for surgery and what do you need to consider?**

A Working with the surgical team, the anaesthetist coordinated a safe transfer to the operating table. Malcolm was in supine position with both arms extended on arm boards. The team ensured that the spinal column and hips were in alignment, and the arms were positioned at an angle of less than 90° to prevent risk of nerve damage to the brachial plexus, ulnar and other superficial nerves in the arm (AfPP, 2011). Other pressure areas were protected, including the occiput on a pillow, the knees were not hyperextended, and gel heel pads were used to reduce pressure on the heel and calf (AfPP, 2011). During the intraoperative phase the surgeon may request Trendelenburg or reverse Trendelenburg to improve surgical access, therefore additional table attachments at the shoulders were used to ensure that patient movement was minimal. The use of a gel pressure-relieving mattress also assists with minimising movement of the patient.

9 **Why might it be necessary to remove some of Malcolm's body hair?**

A Malcolm was moderately hairy so clippers were used to remove hair from the abdomen and also an area of the right thigh (necessary for safe placement of the diathermy electrode). This was performed immediately prior to surgery to reduce the risk of surgical site infection (SSI) (AfPP, 2011). A visual check was made to ensure that Malcolm was not touching any metal part of the operating table, to prevent diathermy burns (AfPP, 2011). The return electrode (plate) was placed on the prepared right thigh with no evidence of previous surgery or other scar tissue, and away from bony prominences (AfPP, 2011).

10 **What interventions are required prior to the commencement of surgery?**

A In order to maintain patient safety, a time out (NPSA, 2010) was instigated by the surgeon with a member of the circulating team, the anaesthetist and the scrub practitioner. Once all of these essential checks had been completed, a trained practitioner inserted a urinary catheter as a result of the TEA, but also to monitor urinary output and prevent retention (Gustafsson *et al.,* 2013). The surgical site was prepared with chlorhexidine alcohol to reduce the risk of SSIs (AfPP, 2011), and disposable drapes were applied by the surgeon and first assistant to establish the sterile field, further reducing the risk of SSIs (AfPP, 2011).

11 **What will the surgical procedure involve?**

A A transverse incision was made to the skin rather than a midline incision, as evidence suggests that this approach causes less postoperative pain offering a good cosmetic result (ERPP, 2010), which may result in reduced anxiety in terms of altered body image. The assessment of the surgeon resulted in the decision to perform an open procedure, however within the ERP laparoscopic procedures are preferred because they are less invasive and lead to a faster recovery (ERPP, 2010; Gustafsson et al., 2013).

A right hemicolectomy will remove the ascending colon, as well as the first part of the transverse colon, caecum and part of the terminal ileum and mesentery (Rothrock, 2011). The mesentery is incised at the terminal ileum and the transverse colon where the resection will be done, and with blunt dissection the vessels are clamped, cut and tied. Larger vessels may be transfixed with a suture to ensure they do not slip off the vessels. At this stage the surgeon will use crushing bowel clamps on the transverse colon and ileum, and non-crushing bowel clamps on the ileum and trans-verse colon. A scalpel is used to divide the affected bowel and provide the scrub practitioner with the specimen (Rothrock, 2011). The scrub practitioner confirmed with the surgeon the nature of the specimen and whether it could be placed in a pot for formalin (formaldehyde) to be added. The properties of formalin fix the specimen, preventing cell deterioration. This will assist the pathologist in determining whether the cells are normal or cancerous (Cancer Research UK, 2014b). The specimen was provided to the circulating practitioner and a label attached with all essential details included; this was shown to the scrub practitioner, logged in the specimen book and the specimen form completed (AfPP, 2011).

The surgeon performed a side-to-side anastomosis by inserting the linear stapler into the ileum and transverse colon, and followed this by using a further linear stapler to close the two stumps (Rothrock, 2011).

12   How would homeostasis be maintained throughout the procedure?

A   Maintaining normothermia of >36°C has been shown to improve postoperative recov-ery (Gustafsson et al., 2013); this was achieved by warming IV fluids and applying a forced air warming blanket throughout the duration of the perioperative experience (Allman and Wilson, 2011; Gustafsson et al., 2013).

An oesophageal Doppler was used to monitor cardiac output (Allman and Wilson, 2011) and, within the ERP, to provide an opportunity for goal-directed fluid therapy. This allowed the anaesthetist to administer enough IV fluids to maintain adequate cardiac output without excess fluid accumulation in the tissues leading to a longer period of recovery. The effects of TEA may lead to hypotension, however within the ERP it is important that these are managed with vasopressors such as ephedrine rather than increased IV fluids (Gustafsson et al., 2013). Mechanical bowel prepara-tion should also be avoided as this will lead to dehydration (ERPP, 2010).

13   What care interventions would Malcolm require in the post-anaesthetic care unit (PACU?)

A   Malcolm was extubated under light anaesthesia to reduce the risk of airway complica-tions in theatre, and a detailed handover from the anaesthetist and the scrub practi-tioner was provided to the recovery practitioner. Malcolm was prescribed oxygen for the first 48 hours to ensure his saturation stayed above 95%, and his urine output was monitored hourly for up to 48 hours (Allman and Wilson, 2011). He received routine monitoring for an extended period in the PACU (ERPP, 2010) and a forced air warming blanket was used to maintain normothermia prior to discharge to the ward. The TEA was set up to provide low-dose local anaesthesia and opioids to provide adequate analgesia for 72 hours to help reduce the risk of ileus (Gustafsson *et al.*, 2013); other analgesics were also prescribed, including paracetamol and ibuprofen (ERPP, 2010).

14 **What does the postoperative rehabilitation phase of the enhanced recovery programme involve?**

A On an ERP Malcolm was supported to mobilise as early as possible as this has been shown to reduce the risk of chest infections and VTEs, and promotes the return of normal intestinal function (ERPP, 2010). To reduce the risk of a urinary tract infection (UTI) the catheter was removed on the second day following surgery (ERPP, 2010; Gustafsson *et al.*, 2013). The stoma nurse visited Malcolm to provide ongoing support with the ileostomy, improving Malcolm's confidence to manage this once discharged home (ERPP, 2010). A one-piece stoma bag was placed around the stoma, with a clear collection bag allowing for immediate postoperative monitoring. The stoma nurse discussed the possibility of alternatives for use at home including a two-piece stoma bag with a flanged adhesive base that sits around the stoma with a changeable bag.

Daily targets were set for Malcolm based on the key elements of the ERP, including early mobilisation, adequately managing his pain, and return to eating and drinking (White and Rivett, 2012). These were set from the day of surgery to the previously agreed discharge date (set at the preoperative visit), five days later. Malcolm was provided with a diary of daily goals including space to write down what he had achieved (White and Rivett, 2012). The daily goals empowered Malcolm to be actively involved in his own recovery and provided him with a record of his progress. Family members were encouraged to assist Malcolm with his daily goals to aid his recovery. Mobilisation was encouraged from the day of surgery, including sitting in the chair for short periods of time. Malcolm was encouraged to walk for longer distances and sit out of bed for longer periods of time, and asked to record his achievements.

On the day of surgery fluid intake was encouraged, followed by food and drink over the days that followed. Malcolm recorded his daily goals in the diary and, once he was able to tolerate both food and drink, the urinary catheter and his intravenous drip were removed, aiding his continued mobilisation and providing the nutritional requirements to support his recovery. Adequate pain management needs constant monitoring at this stage to ensure that it aids in Malcolm's mobilisation and his long-term recovery.

Stop and think

We have explored the rehabilitation phase of the enhanced recovery programme, which aims to improve Malcolm's physical recovery. However, take a moment to reflect upon how you think Malcolm may be feeling at this stage – do you think he will be relieved or perhaps have new concerns? How can you support him most effectively during this period?

15 **What ongoing support do you think Malcolm may require for his continued recovery?**

A Integral to a successful ERP, Malcolm was provided with contact information to improve his confidence following discharge that there were support services in place once he was at home (ERPP, 2010; White and Rivett, 2012). Primary care staff were involved in the preoperative planning of Malcolm's ERP and it is important for them to be contacted with all relevant information to continue to support Malcolm during rehabilitation and onwards to the reversal of his ileostomy.

Other considerations may include:

- altered body image, and the potential impact upon his relationship
- his family
- management of ileostomy
  - nutrition and diet
  - stoma care and collection bag changes
- independence
  - getting to and from the toilet at home
  - getting in and out of bed
- analgesia
- preparing for the reversal of ileostomy
- living with the diagnosis of cancer
- his farm, which is his livelihood.

REFERENCES AND FURTHER READING

Allman, K.G. and Wilson, I.H. (eds) (2011) *Oxford Handbook of Anaesthesia* (3rd edn). Oxford: Oxford University Press.

Association for Perioperative Practice (AfPP) (2011) *Standards and Recommendations for Safe Perioperative Practice*. Harrogate: Association for Perioperative Practice.

Cancer Research UK (2014a) Bowel cancer symptoms. Available online at: www.cancerresearchuk. org/cancer-help/type/bowel-cancer/about/bowel-cancer-symptoms#symptoms (accessed 19 August 2015).

Cancer Research UK (2014b) Bowel cancer (colorectal cancer). Available online at: www.cancerresearchuk.org/cancer-help/type/bowel-cancer (accessed 19 August 2015).

Department of Health (DH) (2009) Reference guide to consent for examination or treatment (2nd edn). Available online at: www.gov.uk/government/uploads/system/uploads/attachment_data/file/138296/dh_103653__1_.pdf (accessed 19 August 2015).

Enhanced Recovery Partnership Programme (ERPP) (2010) *Delivering Enhanced Recovery: Helping Patients to get Better Sooner after Surgery*. London: Crown Copyright.

Gustafsson, U.O., Scott, M.J., Schwenk, W., Demartines, N., Roulin, D., Francis, N., McNaught, C.E., MacFie, J., Liberman, A.S., Soop, M., Hill, A., Kennedy, R.H., Lobo, D.N., Fearon, K. and Ljungqvist, O. (2013) Guidelines for perioperative care in elective colonic surgery: Enhanced Recovery After Surgery (ERAS) Society recommendations. *World Journal of Surgery*, **37**(2): 259–284.

National Patient Safety Agency (NPSA) (2010) *How to Guide: 5 Steps to Safer Surgery*. London: NPSA.

Rothrock, J.C. (2011) *Alexander's Care of the Patient in Surgery* (14th edn). St Louis, MO: Elsevier Mosby.

White, L. and Rivett, K. (2012) *Guidelines for Patients Undergoing Surgery as Part of an Enhanced Recovery Programme (ERP)*. London: Royal College of Anaesthetists.

Hypospadias: the care of James Miller

Karen Evans

INTRODUCTION AND LEARNING OUTCOMES

Hypospadias is a non-hereditary, congenital condition and refers to the urethral meatus located below where expected. Alternatively, if the urethral opening is above the expected site, it is known as epispadias. Relatively common in boys, affecting approximately 1:300, it is much rarer in girls, affecting approximately 1:500,000.

In boys with the condition, more than 80% will have a distal urethral opening anywhere from the mid-shaft to the glans penis; the less common proximal hypospadias results in urethral openings anywhere from the mid-shaft, in or behind the scrotum. There are two associated deformities that can occur: downward curvature of the penis (chordee) and incomplete foreskin development, which can be the primary indication of the condition at birth.

By the end of this case study you will be able to:

- explain how the principles of paediatric perioperative care can be applied to a child undergoing hypospadias repair
- describe how child health and well-being can be promoted in the perioperative environment
- discuss how family-centred care can be implemented through a child's journey, to promote the well-being of both the child and their carer(s).

Case outline

James Miller, aged ten months, was diagnosed with a distal hypospadias defect during routine post-natal checks, and has been regularly reviewed by the paediatric plastic surgeon and urologist since his diagnosis. He lives with his mother, Jane, in a two-bedroom flat in the city centre. James's father is not present in his life, and Jane has not heard from him since before James was born. Although her family lives abroad, Jane has a supportive local network of friends. She works part-time as a secretary and while she is at work James has a childminder who lives nearby and she reports he is happily settled there.

Jane indicates that James is a happy, sociable baby and that, apart from the recommended vaccination programme, he has been fit and well since birth. He is still breastfeeding in the morning and evening, but takes a bottle happily during the day.

Although James is at the younger age limit for this surgery, both Jane and the surgeon have agreed that it is appropriate. Shared decision making is fundamental to the principles of caring for children and their carers, and the active participation of family/carers in providing care for the child is the basis for family-centred care and key to good outcomes regardless of setting (Department of Health (DH), 2004). The decision was based on several factors, as follows.

- Memory formation is limited in this age group, so James is less likely to be psychologically affected by the experience of surgery or recovery at this stage, e.g. if James were potty trained it could be difficult for him to reconcile his new-found independence with a return to nappies for his postoperative care.
- He is increasingly physically active, potentially making later wound management problematic as increased physicality, which is still uncoordinated, could cause wound trauma.
- Jane wishes to emigrate to join her family, but wants this surgeon to undertake the procedure; she feels they have a good, trusting relationship, which is important (DH, 2004).
- Jane has researched the condition extensively and feels that, psychologically, it is important for James to have surgery before becoming genitally aware.
- Position of the urethra is at the base of the glans penis. Children requiring more complex multistage repairs may need to wait until enough tissue is available to form the required grafts. However, Jane is aware that, if a single-stage repair is not possible during this surgery, James's foreskin will be retained for further surgical intervention in the future.
- Evidence suggests that catheterisation causes less bladder spasm in infants, reducing distress, and reducing the risk of urine bypassing the catheter and causing fistula formation along the wound tract.

James was listed for a day surgery procedure in the local specialist paediatric unit, and the surgeon gained surgical consent from Jane in the outpatients department (OPD). Specialised information leaflets, containing information about the day surgery pathway, procedure, pre-admission instructions and postoperative care required, were given to Jane. Additional information on how to access further electronic resources was made available; this element of information giving is now seen as best practice (Royal College of Surgeons (RCS), 2013).

There is a well-established evidence base supporting preoperative visiting for children and their families, and its value in psychological preparation, however this is not offered locally for operational and economic reasons and, instead, a telephone number is provided to allow parents to discuss any aspects of care, ask questions or arrange discussion with the appropriate clinician (RCS, 2013).

1   **What considerations are important as part of the preoperative preparation and assessment process prior to hospital admission?**

A   Local practice is to preoperatively screen ASA 1 paediatric day surgery patients by telephone. If alerts are raised during this process then a face-to-face appointment will be made. No tests are carried out routinely on this group of patients (Royal College of Anaesthetists (RCoA), 2014), but in this case perioperative screening was carried out via the telephone by the paediatric pre-assessment nurse, including family medical history as well as that relating directly to James. Additional factors considered were as follows.

- Gestational age at birth: this impacts directly on suitability for day surgery as pre-term babies can have increased risks of postoperative respiratory complications.
- Social circumstances: to ensure that James will be discharged to the care of his mother and that arrangements have been made to care for him during his recovery in an appropriate environment. Jane has taken a fortnight off work to care for James during the early recovery stages and her childminder will then provide care for him. Jane is happy that she will be able to show the childminder what to do – if not, she will contact the nurses at her local GP surgery.
- Discharge criteria: including journey time from hospital in case of complications, telephone access and transportation options.

Jane was encouraged to ask questions about any aspects of the information she had been given. She was also reminded of clothes, food/milk, special toys, etc., that James may need – for example, clean old pyjamas with a buttoned top as he would remain in these for his anaesthetic and be re-dressed postoperatively. He is very fond of his 'pig' teddy and Jane has requested that this accompany him to both the operating theatre (OT) and post-anaesthetic care unit (PACU).

James's care pathway was made available to the OT and PACU teams for review the day prior to admission.

2   **What should you consider when admitting James and his mother to the unit?**

A   On admission James and Jane were welcomed and orientated to the unit. The play therapy team leads this aspect of the process, and ensures that age-appropriate toys are available, and that both James and Jane have a relaxed introduction. This is essential to minimise admission anxiety; children – in particular infants – respond to parental anxiety and this, combined with stress caused by hospitalisation, can have a negative impact on their experience and recovery. Anxiety and poor experiences can affect this and subsequent admissions; examples include increased incidence of emergence delirium, increased pain and ongoing behavioural changes, which can last long after the admission, e.g. bedwetting and separation anxiety (Tan, 2010; O'Sullivan and Wong, 2013).

3   **Which observations and assessments would be performed on admission and what would you expect for a child of this age?**

A   Routine observations were carried out as per local protocols, and James's physical parameters were within expected ranges for this age group (Table 16.1).

Table 16.1 Routine observation results for James

	Temperature	Heart rate	Respiratory rate	Systolic blood pressure	Diastolic blood pressure
Expected range*	36.5–37.5°C	80–120 bpm	25–40 breaths/ minute	80–100 mmHg	50–65 mmHg
James's baseline	36.9°C	106	28	95 mmHg	55 mmHg

* Consensus gained from multiple sources for an infant 6–12 months

- *Level of consciousness*: James was awake, alert and calmly playing with some toys.
- *Airway and breathing*: manual, visual and auditory checks were undertaken, to obtain a respiratory rate, to listen for abnormal expiratory/inspiratory sounds and to observe any indicators of respiratory distress such as accessory muscle use or intercostal/subcostal recession. Deviations from the 'norm' would indicate a degree of respiratory distress. SpO$_2$ readings were also taken. These observations provide a baseline and can identify previously undetected upper respiratory tract infection, a high risk for perioperative respiratory complications. Any signs of infection would mean postponement of the surgery.
- *Circulation*: a manual pulse was taken from the dorsalis pedis, as James seemed to tolerate this better than the radial or other sites; this was also correlated with the SpO$_2$ monitor reading. It is best practice to obtain a manual pulse, allowing the practitioner to assess rhythm and amplitude; the reading should be carried out for a full 60 seconds, ensuring the reading accurately reflects heart rate.
- *Blood pressure*: as James was compliant, blood pressure (BP) was obtained as per recommendations (Royal College of Surgeons (RCoS), 2013). It can be difficult to auscultate a BP on a small child, despite good technique and a placid child, and they may not tolerate having bilateral readings taken to establish which arm provides the higher reading. Therefore, as a dominant hand may not yet be apparent, statistics would suggest that the right arm is used initially, although other sites can be used such as the lower limbs. Regardless of limb selected, care must be taken to ensure that there is approximately 80% cuff coverage to promote accuracy – too small leads to overestimation and too large to underestimation.
- *Disability and exposure*: James was weighed, in his pyjamas and a dry nappy, at 10 kg putting him between the 50th and 75th centile for his age. It was confirmed that James had been starved appropriately, i.e. last breastfed four hours prior to anaesthesia, with clear oral fluids permitted up to two hours before. Had James been fed on cows' or artificial formula milk, his last feed time would have been six hours prior to surgery, allowing for the differences in gastric emptying time followed by the same clear fluid regime.

Visual skin integrity checks were also made, in particular of James's skin under the nappy to ensure that the tissue around the operation site did not show signs of rash or tissue damage, which could have impaired wound healing.

A urinalysis dipstick was used to check urine in a wet nappy. While not definitive, this crude method could identify overt indications of a urinary tract infection (UTI), such as proteins and blood. If signs of UTI had been present, surgery may have been postponed, as a urinary catheter is required for a minimum of two weeks postoperatively. Had a more accurate result been needed, a collection bag would have been given to Jane by the OPD team. This bag has an adherent ring placed over the genitalia to collect a sample for testing via the GP surgery.

Temperature was obtained using an infrared tympanic thermometer; alternatively, axillary temperature could have been obtained using an electronic thermometer probe. Chemical dot thermometers are not used locally due to the risk of reaction when used repeatedly.

If James had been distressed during these essential checks, the play therapist would have been alerted to provide distraction activities. Discharge arrangements were confirmed and the preoperative checklist was completed. Two computer-generated wristbands were applied – one to James's left wrist and one to his right ankle – ensuring that access should be possible at every stage of his journey. A topical local anaesthetic cream was not applied as James would be having a gas induction.

4   **What do you think are the key considerations that the anaesthetist will discuss as part of the plan for anaesthetic management?**

A   The anaesthetist met with Jane and James to review the information obtained during preoperative assessment, and to discuss the plans he had for anaesthetic management, as follows.

- Inhalational induction: relatively atraumatic for James, as he can sit on Jane's lap and his intravenous cannula can be inserted after induction when the vasodilatory effects of the volatile agent will assist with placement of the cannula.
- Laryngeal mask airway: this supraglottic airway is easily inserted and has demonstrated a reduction in postoperative respiratory and airway complications.
- Caudal block: to provide intra- and postoperative analgesia for James. Complication rates are low and these blocks demonstrate a high level of success in managing postoperative pain.
- Simple analgesia: a low-risk multimodal analgesic approach, which helps avoid opioid usage. Opioids increase the incidence of respiratory depression, postoperative nausea and vomiting (PONV) and sedation.
- Anti-emetic: to reduce incidence of PONV. PONV causes distress to patients, and can prolong recovery and length of stay.
- Intravenous fluid replacement: to prevent dehydration, and reduce the risk of PONV and the potential distress of feeling thirsty.

Verbal consent was obtained and Jane was encouraged to ask any questions she might have about the anaesthetic (Association of Anaesthetists of Great Britain and Ireland (AAGBI), 2010).

5 **What preparation of the theatre environment is necessary prior to James arriving for surgery?**

A Routine safety and quality checks on cleanliness, equipment and environment were undertaken prior to the list commencement. Theatre ambient temperature was increased to 23°C, to compensate for any radiating heat loss.

6 **What do you think needs to be discussed as part of the team brief for this case?**

A James was first on the list, to minimise his starvation time as hunger can make small children additionally distressed (Shields, 2010). The anaesthetist described his anaesthetic plan and the surgeon requested a hypospadias set, alongside his other surgical requirements. This set contains the following specific instruments.

- Castroviejo needle holder: locking mechanism to ensure controlled grip; holds fine needles for delicate tissue closure.
- Barron knife handle: octagonal, allowing precise fingertip control of depth and course; can also be rotated if required.
- Bowman probes and Dittel urethral bougies (8 CH–6 CH); for dilation of urethra or tracking of false channels.
- Skin hooks: Kilner Catspaw and Gillies.
- Urinary catheter: 6 and 8 FG available.
- Marker pens and ruler: marking graft site(s) and measuring distance from existing site to that desired and urethral length.

Roles and emergency roles were agreed, although no problems were anticipated. Support for Jane, to escort her from the anaesthetic room to the parents' waiting area and ensure that she was not distressed, was allocated to a member of the team, who went to the waiting area to introduce herself to Jane and James. This strategy aims to help reduce 'stranger anxiety' for James (Shields, 2010) and allow Jane a familiar face to focus on when requested to leave the anaesthetic room.

7 **How would you care for James and engage Jane in his care at induction of anaesthesia?**

A Jane, James and 'pig' were collected from the waiting room. Jane was encouraged to sit comfortably in a chair with James on her lap, acting as secure reassurance for James (Shields, 2010; O'Sullivan and Wong, 2013). James looked bewildered by the new faces and anaesthetic room, even though staff numbers were kept to a minimum, voices kept low and calm, and the anaesthetic room was 'child-friendly' with colourful pictures and contemporary cartoon figures decorating the space (Tan, 2010; RCoA, 2014). The sign-in process commenced.

Bubbles were used as a distraction while SpO_2 monitoring was applied in the form of an adherent finger wrap. Once secured, a face mask was held close to James's face, commencing the inhalational induction process. Sevoflurane, oxygen (O_2) and nitrous oxide (N_2O) were delivered using a T-piece system. Sevoflurane is a pleasant-smelling volatile agent with a rapid onset and fast recovery time; N_2O

increases the speed and depth of anaesthesia, while O_2 maintains tissue oxygenation. This combination would also be used to maintain anaesthesia during the procedure.

As James started to drift off to sleep, the anaesthetist applied the mask completely over his mouth and nose. Once satisfied that James was asleep he was placed gently on the operating trolley and Jane was asked to leave after giving him a kiss. Jane was escorted to the parents' waiting area.

8   **Once James is asleep and Jane has left the anaesthetic room, what anaesthetic care interventions will be undertaken?**

A   Additional monitoring in the form of electrocardiography, blood pressure and skin temperature sensors were applied, unbuttoning or removing James's pyjamas as required, and baseline anaesthetic observations obtained. Care was taken to minimise exposure and reduce inadvertent heat loss.

The anaesthetic practitioner inserted and secured a 22G cannula into the dorsum of James's right hand. In infants, vein size rather than flow rate tends to dictate cannula size with the largest possible being inserted. If this is not adequate to allow rapid correction of fluid imbalance – for example, in a bleeding child – then an additional cannula would be inserted.

An intravenous (IV) fluid maintenance infusion of Hartmann's solution was commenced. Only isotonic solutions of Hartmann's solution and sodium chloride 0.9% are routinely used within the local trust, because of the increased risk of hyponatraemia in the paediatric patient. Hypotonic solutions exert less osmotic pressure on cell membranes, encouraging fluid shifts from the intravascular space to the intracellular and interstitial spaces. Normal physiological response would be to inhibit anti-diuretic hormone (ADH) production, increasing urinary output. However, increased secretion of ADH can be triggered by many factors, which are particularly pertinent to the perioperative setting (e.g. pain, anxiety, PONV). Normal responses are inhibited, water is retained and extracellular volume becomes expanded, with consequences including acute cerebral oedema and neurological injury. It is of note that some isotonic fluids, when metabolised, become hypotonic, e.g. 5% dextrose.

A micro burette system was utilised. This delivers 60 drops/ml ensuring internal vascular pressure is minimised. These systems have an additional safety feature: the volume chamber holds one hour's worth of IV fluid for administration, ensuring that any inadvertent changes to flow will restrict the volume of fluid infused.

A laryngeal mask airway (LMA), size 1.5, was inserted and, once secured, was connected to the T-piece, allowing spontaneous breathing of the gas mixture. Appropriately sized Robertshaw blades, laryngoscope handles and a range of endotracheal tubes were available should this have been unsuccessful.

James's nappy was removed and he was positioned laterally with hips flexed to 90°, allowing optimal access for the caudal block. Skin preparation was applied and, while this was drying, 'Stop before you block' was undertaken. The anaesthetist delivered an injection of levobupivacaine and clonidine, aseptically. Levobupivacaine was used as it reduces motor blockade, which can be distressing for the younger child. As the anaesthetist wished to avoid the use of opiates, particularly as James was a day surgery case, clonidine was added to prolong analgesic effect, approximately doubling block efficacy. An alternative, if caudal blockade was unsuccessful, would be an intraoperative penile block. IV paracetamol 7.5 mg/kg was given using a syringe; this practice has been adopted since 2010 safety notices alerted the team to the risks of infusing paracetamol to paediatric patients using an IV line. IV ondansetron was administered. Eye protection was applied.

9   How will James's temperature be maintained intraoperatively?

A   James was placed supine on the operating trolley, on top of an underbody forced air warming blanket, which would be calibrated according to his temperature measurements and transferred into theatre. Relatively large surface area to body mass ratios and immature thermoregulatory responses mean that children need careful management to prevent inadvertent perioperative hypothermia; considerations are environmental (radiation, evaporation, convection and conduction), decreased metabolic activity and cooling effects of drug administration.

10   What will the surgical process involve for this case?

A   Once the anaesthetist was happy that it was safe to proceed, the 'time out' process was completed. Skin preparation was performed and surgical drapes applied: one small drape under his bottom and a fenestrated drape applied to his operative site.

A tubularised incised plate (TIP) urethroplasty was undertaken to create a slit-like meatus at the tip of the glans penis (Stone, 2008). The penis was de-gloved and an artificial erection created, to assess for undetected chordee. This was not evident. The 'wings' of the glans penis were then excised from the urethral plate, which was then tubularised and measurements taken to check for adequate length; then it was rolled over a 6FG Foley urinary catheter and a layered closure completed with polyglactin sutures. A dartos pedicle flap, taken from the dorsal foreskin, was used to cover the repair. Glanular wings and remaining tissue were closed on the midline using polyglactin sutures. Had there been excessive blood loss, a Foley catheter would have been used to create a penile tourniquet, however blood loss was managed with bipolar diathermy. This technique was used as it does not require a return pad or plate, minimising risk from poor contact or allergic reaction.

The circumcision procedure was completed and closed using cyanoacrylate glue. This closure technique is rapidly applied with comparable cosmetic results to suturing; it also has the benefits of forming a barrier layer and does not require removal. A petroleum gauze and non-adherent gauze dressing were applied and secured with hypoallergenic tape. Had a circumcision not been undertaken, a silastic foam dressing would have been used to provide additional support for the penis. A double-nappy technique was then used; a small hole was formed in the inner nappy to allow the distal end of the catheter to be threaded through into the outer, allowing for free drainage of urine while keeping the wound site dry.

James's skin was checked for any signs of tissue damage, before he was re-dressed in his pyjamas. His warming blanket was left in situ, in case required for temperature management in the post-anaesthetic care unit (PACU). James was positioned left laterally, supported by pillows, warmed blankets applied and 'pig' tucked in beside him. Eye protection was removed. The surgical 'sign out' was then completed prior to transfer to the PACU.

11   **What assessment and care would James initially require during first-stage recovery in the PACU?**

A   James was received into first-stage recovery, and rapid assessments carried out prior to the commencement of anaesthetic and surgical handover, as follows.

- Level of consciousness: James was unconscious.
- Airway and breathing: airway secured with an untied LMA. Manual, visual and auditory checks were undertaken. James was spontaneously breathing, with a regular rate of 25 breaths/minute and good depth of respiration. No indicators of respiratory distress were noted. SpO_2 100% on 40% O_2, and no evidence of central or peripheral cyanosis.
- Circulation: pulse was within expected parameters (see Table 16.1) at 100 bpm.

Blood pressure is not normally undertaken in the PACU unless requested. In children, circulation is driven by heart rate rather than circulating volume, so a fall in BP is a late sign of shock and heart rate is a better indicator of distress.

Handover was taken and postoperative care confirmed by the PACU practitioner. James was observed to be moving quickly through the reversing stages of anaesthesia – an advantage of the sevoflurane and desirable for day surgery patients (Hatfield, 2014). James was carefully observed for return of his protective reflexes and, shortly after admission to the PACU, he roused, coughed and expelled his LMA. Gentle suction was applied to the visible oropharynx to clear secretions that had accumulated during the procedure. Sevoflurane can cause increased risks of emergence delirium postoperatively, and staff were monitoring for signs of this on emergence.

James snuggled back into the pillows and a full assessment was carried out. While this was occurring a member of staff went to collect Jane from the parents' waiting room. As soon as practicable, a child and their carer should be reunited as this means familiar loved faces for the child to wake up to, leading to a reduction in undesirable distress and anxiety for both (Tan, 2010; O'Sullivan and Wong, 2013; Hatfield, 2014).

- Level of consciousness: James was rousable to gentle touch.
- Airway and breathing: spontaneously breathing, good rate and depth. No signs of cyanosis.
- Circulation: pulse within expected parameters, capillary refill < 2 seconds.
- Disability and exposure: nappies left intact but checks made for any signs of haemorrhage around the leg- and waistbands, plus observation for signs of discolouring to the nappies. The IV infusion and site were checked for patency and flow rate as this can change depending on limb position, height of the infusion bag, etc. A light, temporary bandage was applied, until James started oral fluids, at which stage the IV infusion would be discontinued.

While self-report is seen as the gold standard for pain assessment, in infants of James's age communication can be difficult. A behavioural tool was used, based on the FLACCs tool (Face, Legs, Activity, Cry and Consolability), applying a score to observed behaviours to achieve a pain assessment. Where possible, carers should be involved in this process as they can recognise and distinguish behavioural cues such as hunger or fear from pain and distress responses.

- Temperature: within expected range.

Jane arrived and was encouraged to sit with James while he woke up. She explained that this was his normal nap time and he normally slept heavily. With this in mind, and in view of the fact that his five-minutely observations were stable, James was moved to second stage.

12 **How would you continue to care for James in the second stage of recovery?**

A Observations continued every 15 minutes and James remained stable. Once he had awoken from his sleep, he was irritable and 'grumpy'. He was lifted on to Jane's lap, allowing her to feed him. Following this he became bright and happy, playing with 'pig' and other toys from the unit. His IV infusion was discontinued and they were taken through to third stage.

13 **What information do you think it is important to give Jane in the third stage of recovery as you start to plan for James to be discharged?**

A Here Jane was given the postoperative instruction sheets containing information on the following.

- Avoidance of physical activity where trauma could be caused inadvertently, e.g. sit-on toys.
- Recommendations for increased oral intake, to reduce risks of a urinary tract infection.
- Removal of the penile dressings, which should be left for three days, unless soiled by faeces, to optimise wound healing.
- Maintenance of skin hygiene and monitoring for signs of infection in/around the wound.
- Catheter care, remaining in situ for ten days postoperatively until OPD review.
- Management of the double nappy system, demonstrated with an outer nappy change.
- Pain management once the analgesic effect of the caudal had worn off – regular administration of oral paracetamol suspension for five days.
- If bladder spasms from the catheter are causing pain and discomfort, Jane was advised to contact the unit, where an anti-spasmodic, oxybutynin, would be prescribed to relieve this.

Although the specific immediate postoperative risks were discussed when Jane gave her consent, these were reiterated, with explanation of how to identify and take appropriate action – specifically the risks of bleeding, infection – both wound and urinary – blocked catheter or bladder spasm causing urine to bypass the catheter. At each point Jane was encouraged to ask questions and her understanding was confirmed. Jane was also given the 24-hour helpline number in case she wished to discuss any concerns, had queries or just needed reassurance.

James had taken oral fluids and nutrition, passed urine via the catheter into the outer nappy, showed no sign of pain or nausea, and was mobilising around the unit, albeit a little gingerly due to the bulk of his nappy. His IV cannula was removed, and Jane and James were ready for discharge home.

14 **What longer-term follow up do you think James will require?**

A The aim of James's surgery is to allow normal urinary and sexual function, and give a natural appearance to his penis as it develops. He will be followed up until he reaches sexual maturity to check for urethral stenosis, development of undetected chordee, urethral fistula formation (affects about 1:10), ability to gain an erection and for any developing psychological issues experienced as he matures.

Stop and think

Having completed this case study, reflect upon the holistic care considerations and the patient experience of both the paediatric patient and their parent/carer. Try to consider the following key learning points and think about how you could embed them within your own practice:

- Family-centred care empowers both child and carer(s).
- Age-appropriate communication develops therapeutic relationships with children.
- Psychological development affects the child's experience.
- Physical and physiological development alters care delivery.
- Involve specialists to support care delivery, and enhance child and family experience, e.g. play therapists, hospital school staff.
- The care experience can have long-lasting negative effects on children.

REFERENCES AND FURTHER READING

Association of Anaesthetists of Great Britain and Ireland (AAGBI) (2010) *Pre-operative Assessment and Patient Preparation: The Role of the Anaesthetist.* London: AAGBI.

Department of Health (DH) (2004) *National Service Framework for Children, Young People and Maternity Services.* London: DH Publications.

Hatfield, A. (2014) *The Complete Recovery Room* (5th edn). Oxford: Oxford University Press.

O'Sullivan, M. and Wong, G. (2013), Preinduction techniques to relieve anxiety in children undergoing general anaesthesia. *Continuing Education in Anaesthesia, Critical Care and Pain,* **13**(6): 196–199. Available online at: http://ceaccp.oxfordjournals.org/content/13/6/196.full.pdf (accessed 14 March 2014).

Royal College of Anaesthetists (RCoA) (2014) Guidelines for the provision of anaesthetic services (GPAS) 2014. Available online at: www.rcoa.ac.uk/gpas2014 (accessed 13 March 2014).

Royal College of Nursing (RCN) (2013) Standards for assessing, measuring and monitoring vital signs in infants, children and young people (rev. edn). Available online at: www.rcn.org.uk/__data/assets/pdf_file/0004/114484/003196.pdf (accessed 13 March 2014).

Royal College of Surgeons (RCS) (2013) *Standards for Children's Surgery: Children's Surgical Forum.* London: RCS Publishing.

Shields, L. (ed.) (2010) *Perioperative Care of the Child: A Nursing Manual*. Chichester: Wiley-Blackwell.

Stone, C. (ed.) (2008) *The Evidence for Plastic Surgery*. Shrewsbury: tfm Publishing Limited.

Tan, L. (2010), Anaesthesia for the uncooperative child. *Continuing Education in Anaesthesia, Critical Care and Pain*, **10**(2): 48–52. Available online at: http://ceaccp.oxfordjournals.org/content/10/2/48.short (accessed 13 March 2014).

Insertion of cardiac artery stent: the care of Patricia Stead

Stephen Wordsworth

INTRODUCTION AND LEARNING OUTCOMES

This case study details the perioperative care of a patient undergoing insertion of a coronary artery stent as a result of coronary artery disease (CAD). CAD is demonstrably the most common form of heart disease and results from deposits of atheroscleroma (referred to as plaque), which results in stenosis – or narrowing – of the coronary arteries. NICE (2008) reports that CAD results in around 110,000 deaths annually in England and Wales alone, which is among the highest rate in the world. For patients like Patricia, CAD can result in significant morbidity, leading to a significant reduction in quality of life.

By the end of this case study you will be able to:

- describe the pre-, peri- and postoperative care needs of the patient undergoing a cardiac stent procedure
- establish the rationale of cardiac stenting following a diagnosis of CAD, as well as demonstrate the benefits and drawbacks of the procedure from a patient's perspective
- explain the technique of cardiac stenting and its application in treating stenosis, including its safe and effective use.

Case outline

Patricia Stead is a 65-year-old female. She lives alone following the death of her husband four years ago. Patricia, known to her friends as Pat, has a grown-up daughter who lives some distance from the family home. Up until recently Pat had been in reasonable health, although for the past four years has taken simvastatin 40 mg once per day. Pat had been shocked by the sudden death of her husband following a stroke and her daughter had nagged her to get a check-up, where she was diagnosed with high cholesterol and encouraged to lose weight in order to reduce her body mass index (BMI).

Although Pat had developed a rather sedentary lifestyle she still tried to remain independent and insisted on walking to the local supermarket once a week to do her shopping. On her way home, Pat had to pause, as she often did, at the top of a short hill with her shopping trolley, just to 'catch her breath'. Unlike normal, however, Pat became aware of a tightness in her chest (in line with her sternum). As the pain intensified she described it as if something heavy (a pressure) had been placed on her chest. She began to experience the same feelings on several other occasions, always when engaging in physical activity. Pat describes visiting her daughter a couple of months later, where she 'took a turn for the worse'. She remembers the pain coming on as she walked to the end of the garden, where – in the words of her daughter – she appeared to 'slump to the ground'.

1 **Reflect upon the effectiveness of each stage of Pat's initial care, diagnosis and treatment.**

A Pat remembers the ambulance arriving and then waking up in hospital having been brought into the emergency department (ED), and although she remained conscious throughout she remembers little else about the journey. Pat was given glyceryl trinitrate (GTN) spray and her oxygen saturation (SpO_2) was monitored throughout. Venous access was secured and 2.5 mg diamorphine administered for pain relief.

The earliest pharmacological intervention in the specific treatment of acute coronary syndrome (ACS) is the administration of a single dose of aspirin. It reduces the relative risk of death by 15% and the risk of non-fatal myocardial infarction (MI) by 30% in both the acute phase and in secondary prevention (Theroux et al., 1988). On this occasion Pat was given a 300 mg chewable tablet, to be absorbed through the oral mucosa. Indeed Keenan (2011) reports that oral absorption is preferable in the acute phase due to its rapid onset, and is particularly useful where nausea and vomiting are common.

After an emergency admission, blood tests were taken for full blood count (FBC), renal function, electrolytes, glucose, lipids and clotting. While in the ED Pat was monitored closely, including pulse and blood pressure, heart rate and rhythm, and oxygen saturation. An ED specialist immediately suspected that Pat had experienced an episode of ACS. Rather than using the term myocardial infarction (MI), ACS can refer more accurately to a range of possible cardiac ischaemic episodes.

To establish the specific nature of the ACS, a 12-lead electrocardiogram (ECG) and serial cardiac troponin levels are undertaken as standard diagnostic tests, along with a detailed medical history. The ECG revealed ST elevation, and in conjunction with Pat's medical history, this suggested that she was experiencing stable angina involving acute chest pain of >20 minutes, which is also associated with an ST elevation MI (STEMI). On ECG, ST elevation indicates that a coronary artery has become occluded by a thrombus resulting from an atheromatous plaque, subsequently leading to the death of the heart muscle supplied by the artery concerned.

Although there is regional variation, on average there are around 500 hospitalised episodes per million people each year in the UK (NICE, 2013). In non ST-elevation ACS (NSTE-ACS), patients also present with acute chest pain but without persistent ST-segment elevation. NICE (2010a) best practice guidelines indicate that in NSTE the prognosis can be poor, especially in the absence of early intervention, which can lead to additional cardiovascular events including myocardial infarction, stroke and the need for repeat revascularisation, or even death.

The protein troponin is not normally found in blood serum and is released only after some degree of myocardial necrosis has occurred. Therefore, as a diagnostic tool, troponin is a specific and sensitive indicator of cardiac damage, which is normally detectable within 3–12 hours, peaking at 24–48 hours after the onset of chest pain (NICE, 2010b). Damage to the myocardium itself may not be detectable until six hours later. Bloods were taken from Pat on admission to the ED and confirmed the presence of troponin. The same test was then scheduled to be repeated after 12 hours. Other tests for the presence of further cardiac enzymes were carried out, including detection of creatine kinase (CK-MB) found mainly in cardiac muscle, and which becomes raised within 3–12 hours, reaching a peak within 24 hours of the onset of the ACS. A further enzyme, myoglobin, is released from damaged cardiac muscle more rapidly than both troponin and creatine kinase, and in Pat's case was found to be present within two hours of the myocardial infarct and one hour after admission to hospital.

A detailed medical history revealed that Pat had been experiencing mild angina for a number of months but had put it down to heartburn and indigestion. Over the past couple of weeks Pat had experienced increasing shortness of breath, accompanied by angina, whose onset had become more frequent and lasted longer on her regular walk home from the shops. While visiting her daughter Pat had felt dizzy and felt the 'pain becoming more intense', but thought that 'it would go away in time and went to get some fresh air'.

Stop and think

Consider how a thorough clinical history can lead to an accurate diagnosis of acute coronary syndrome.

- Onset: patient experiences sudden onset of chest pain and/or shortness of breath, often preceded by shorter episodes of discomfort either at rest or on exertion.
- Location: pain located in centre or upper chest, radiating into the neck, throat or jaw, and into the upper arms.
- Duration: establish the duration and initial timing of discomfort; the benefits of therapeutic intervention are time dependent.
- Characteristics: patient describes how it affects them – crushing, suffocating, tightness, heaviness, and dull or deep pain.
- Associated feature: ACS is often associated with shortness of breath. Patients may also look pale, and feel cool and clammy to touch; often accompanied by nausea and vomiting.

- Relieving factors: patients often want to remain still, in the hope that this will reduce the discomfort. There is no positional element to the discomfort, though, and it cannot be reduced.
- Treatments: patients often interpret their symptoms, and use over-the-counter medicines such as antacids or painkillers to relieve their discomfort.

Source: Adapted from Keenan (2011)

Given Pat's history of worsening angina and diagnosis following ECG and cardiac enzyme testing, the treatment of choice is to undergo a non-surgical percutaneous coronary intervention (PCI) as the optimum form of re-vascularisation in patients such as Pat, as an alternative to coronary artery bypass grafting (CABG). PCI involves the widening of the coronary artery, via the insertion of a balloon catheter to dilate the artery. At this point, a metal stent – normally constructed from stainless steel – is placed in the artery in order to keep the lumen of the artery patent.

2   Describe the purpose of PCI re-vascularisation in Pat's treatment?

A   The speed at which PCI re-vascularisation is achieved has been shown to be an important factor in the overall treatment efficacy to perfuse the myocardium and reduce the size of the infarct, thus improving mortality at 30 days, one year and 18 months post-procedure (Keenan, 2011). NICE (2013) best practice guidelines indicate that the 'target window' from 'door to balloon time is 90 minutes'.

Once Pat's condition post-MI had been stabilised in the ED, she was transferred to a specialist cardiac catheterisation lab. The procedure had been fully explained to her by the interventional cardiologist, including the indications, benefits and risks of PCI. Pat gave her informed consent, but expressed her concerns that she would be awake during the procedure and that she felt frightened that she might feel what was happening; she was also 'worried about the wire doing damage to her heart'. Transportation of cardiac patients with ACS is a critical feature of their care, particularly where patients are admitted to district hospital locations but then need to be transferred to a cardiac centre with specialist equipment and staff used to dealing with high-volume PCI. Although this was not necessary for Pat, inter-hospital transportation can increase the risk of morbidity and mortality, and timing, and the preparation and availability of resuscitation equipment, are essential. For a number of ODPs involvement in intra- and inter-hospital transfer may well be a requirement, and they should assure themselves that they have the necessary skills and training to work in this area of extended practice (Wordsworth, 2014). This may involve advanced airway, breathing and circulatory life support and resuscitation, as well as specialist knowledge in ECG interpretation (including 12-lead).

Once in the catheterisation lab Pat was helped into a supine position; she became very anxious and frightened by the presence of the equipment and machinery, and was pleased that she had taken up the option of sedation. Although specialist cardiac nursing staff, along with cardiology medics, usually make up the team, ODPs may find themselves being deployed in the catheterisation lab, particularly during patient transfer and indeed in support of patients in emergency situations, such as those

requiring emergency induction of a GA and neuromuscular blockade to facilitate intubation. It should also be noted that a range of cardiac interventions can also take
place in the operating theatre (OT). A specialist cardiac technician and a radiographer
skilled in angiography imaging technology were also present during Pat's procedure.

Stop and think

What are the benefits of sedation in patients such as Pat who are undergoing a
re-vascularisation procedure?

ECG, BP and pulse oximetry were monitored at all times before, during and after
the procedure, and intravenous access was established in Pat's non-dominant
left hand. An initial bolus dose of propofol, followed by a continuous infusion
was given to the level of 'conscious sedation', to enable Pat to tolerate long
periods of not being able to move. This also helped to reduce her anxiety, but
allowed her to remain able to maintain her own airway and stay responsive to
commands and requests. Propofol, rather than midazolam, is normally preferred
during angioplasty and stenting as it causes less respiratory depression for the
equivalent degree of sedation and anxiolysis. At this point an antithrombotic
drug, in this case 5000 units of heparin as a bolus dose, was given.

---

3 **Reflect upon the need to undertake arterial cannulation.**

A Arterial access in order to perform cardiac catheterisation is normally achieved in
either the femoral artery at the groin, or via the radial artery in the arm or wrist. In
Pat's case the wrist was chosen and has several advantages over femoral access,
including less post-procedural bleeding and bruising (as the artery is smaller, and
more effective pressure can be applied) (Ziakas *et al.*, 2007). Patients are also not
required to lie flat for as long a period of time following radial access.

Prior to catheterisation, an Allen's test was performed to ensure normal circulation
between the radial and ulnar arteries should the radial artery become occluded. The
site of insertion was anaesthetised with 1% lignocaine to provide local anaesthesia
in order to reduce pain and discomfort at the insertion site. The site was also prepared and cleaned aseptically and sterile drapes applied to secure a 'sterile field'. It
is also worth noting that the procedure takes place in a cooled room, so lying still
may lead to a drop in the patient's temperature and staff must remain vigilant regarding the potential for hypothermia.

4 **Describe the surgical technique involved in carrying out a percutaneous coronary
intervention (PCI)?**

A **Cardiac catheterisation and angiography**
With Pat feeling more relaxed, the artery was palpated and a needle entered towards
the arterial pulsation; cannulation was assured when arterial blood was seen to flow
through the needle. With Pat unable to feel anything due to the effects of the local

anaesthetic, a thin, flexible guide wire was introduced with the help of a 'tip deflector' to straighten out any curvature of the guide wire. Both guide wire and needle were then removed to allow a 2.5 mm diameter flexible plastic tube and shield to be advanced over the guide wire and into the artery, in order to act as an introducer for the catheter(s). The sheath sits at the level of the skin and allows a one-way valve to control the insertion of the catheter(s), but prevents blood from escaping.

At this point the catheter, which comprises a long soft plastic tube, was inserted, then 'railroaded' over the guide wire and advanced carefully under x-ray imaging towards the heart. During the advance of the catheter, the cardiologist rotates the device to manipulate the tip carefully through the arterial system and, once at the heart, guides the tip into the opening of the coronary arteries. To assess the coronary arteries and the extent of the stenosis, a contrast medium is injected through the catheter to provide a fluoroscopic (x-ray image), and in Pat's case an image intensifier was used to produce a digital subtraction angiograph (DSA). This involved x-ray detection of the contrast medium, which is subjected to up to 30 exposures per second before being converted into a digital image. At this point the pre-contrast image is 'subtracted' from those taken after the introduction of the contrast, enabling the elimination of bone and tissue that would otherwise be superimposed over the artery in question. The resulting image can then be viewed on a video screen. Image intensification also enables rotation, to allow arterial structures to be viewed from different angles.

During the angiography Pat's heart rate slowed slightly and the cardiologist asked her to cough; this helped to clear the contrast medium from the coronary arteries as this can lead to bradycardia. She also described feeling a 'hot flush', but one that quickly dissipated; the nurse was able to explain that this was normal in many patients.

Percutaneous transluminal coronary angioplasty and stenting
After reviewing the angiogram, only the left anterior descending artery (LAD), which supplies the front of the left side of the heart, and which branches off the left main coronary artery (LMCA), was found to be 65% blocked. NICE (2008) guidelines for the use of a stent require the target artery to be of less than 3 mm calibre, or indeed that the area of stenosis be no longer than 15 mm.

The circumflex artery, which supplies the outer and back of the heart, had very slight narrowing but this was not considered to be clinically significant. In Pat's case the right coronary artery (RCA), which supplies blood to the right atrium and ventricle, as well as the SA (sinoatrial) and AV (atrioventricular) nodes, also proved to be normal. These findings were entirely consistent with a diagnosis of SCAD, which leads to chest-related symptoms as a result of narrowing by more than 50% in the left main coronary artery (ESC, 2013).

At this stage Pat felt sufficiently relaxed and calm to look at the video screen when prompted by the cardiologist, and she could clearly see where the artery narrowed. She was reminded that, when the procedure was explained to her (and consent gained), it would first involve the angiogram, and now the cardiologist explained that he was moving on to the second stage, which included removing the blockage and introducing the stent. With the guide catheter at the origin of the LAD, the guide wire was passed with great care through the artery and across the stenosis to the distal end of the obstruction. It should be noted that the guide catheter also allows for essential and continuous measurement of inter-arterial blood pressure.

Stop and think

List the complications associated with PCI stenting, which are as follows:

- stent thrombosis
- re-stenosis of stent
- acute MI (1%), possibly leading to coronary artery bypass grafting
- stroke
- cardiac tamponade
- systemic bleeding
- allergy to the contrast medium
- nephropathy and complications at the access bleeding and haematoma at the access site
- death.

A separate catheter, in Pat's case with a stent mounted on a balloon, was passed over the guide wire and located under x-ray into position inside the stenosis. At this stage the balloon was inflated, this had the effect of squeezing the atherosclerotic plaque against the arterial wall. After that the thin wire mesh stent was also opened to its maximum diameter as a result of the balloon pressure, thereby acting as a permanent prosthetic lining in order to maintain the arterial patency (ESC, 2013).

During the inflation, patients may experience angina, but in Pat's case she remained pain free throughout; careful attention was also paid to any changes in Pat's ECG, particularly ST-segment depression or elevation should blood flow during angioplasty be restricted. The cardiologist undertook one further balloon inflation to ensure optimal expansion of the stent (Muggenthaler, Singh and Wilkinson, 2008) before the catheter and guide wire were carefully withdrawn. The site of the initial puncture was closed with a suture and a tight dressing applied for two to three hours.

Stent technology
Initial stent technology using bare metal stents (BMS) has now largely been replaced by so-called drug-eluting stents (DES), these are coated with an active drug, usually an immune suppressant, to reduce inflammation. In Pat's case, the antimitotic drug paclitaxel was used, which is intended to reduce cell proliferation. NICE (2008: 6) reports that 'the drug reaches therapeutic concentrations in local tissues only and may not be detectable systemically, thus avoiding systemic adverse effects'.

POST-PROCEDURAL CARE

With the procedure completed Pat was allowed to recover from the effects of the sedation such that she was able to continue to maintain her own airway, and was alert and responding to commands. She was then transferred to the coronary care unit for close monitoring and observation. Staff were careful to observe and note any signs of haemodynamically significant bleeding or cardiac ischaemia evident through the onset of chest pain, and shortness of breath with the possibility of ST-segment changes evident on ECG (Muggenthaler *et al.*, 2008). The catheter insertion site was also observed for signs of a haematoma and, in the case of the radial artery, evidence of peripheral emboli or arterial occlusion.

Stent insertion carries the risk of stent-related thrombosis; patients are therefore required to use aspirin indefinitely as its interruption can lead to a higher risk of further heart attacks and patients should be assessed for their ability to self-medicate in this way (NICE, 2008). Pat was also required to take the anti-platelet drug clopidogrel 75 mg, which NICE (2008) also recommend should be continued for at least 12 months and then reviewed on an individual patient basis.

5 **Reflect upon Pat's long-term recovery.**

A Pat's immediate recovery was uneventful, and after spending the night on the coronary care unit (CCU) she was allowed to go home the following day. Follow-up appointments were made for her to see the cardiologist and her GP. On discharge Pat was provided with information on what to do if she felt any angina pain or if she had concerns about any aspect of her treatment or ongoing care. The importance of taking her anti-platelet medication was stressed and a specialist cardiac nurse spoke to her about lifestyle advice, with the intention of reducing her cardiac risks factors. Although it didn't apply to Pat, patients who have undergone stent insertion following an MI with ST elevation should refrain from driving for four weeks after the procedure (NICE, 2008).

Following the introduction of DES, the long-term outcomes for patients such as Pat have improved significantly, mainly as a result of restoring blood supply to the myocardium, and the avoidance of re-stenosis and subsequent need to repeat the procedure following 'proliferation of smooth muscle within the arterial wall' (usually four to six months post-procedure). NICE (2008) report that the need to carry out further re-vascularisation procedures following DES is less than 5%. Pat immediately reported feeling much better, with the angina now completely gone, such that her quality of life has been significantly improved without the need for further intervention.

REFERENCES AND FURTHER READING

European Society of Cardiology (ESC) (2013) ESC guidelines on the management of stable coronary artery disease. The Taskforce on the Management of Stable Coronary Artery Disease of the European Society of Cardiology. *European Heart Journal*, **34**: 2949–3003.

Keenan, J. (2011) Therapeutic intervention in acute coronary syndromes, in Humphries, M. (ed.) *Nursing the Cardiac Patient*. Chichester: Wiley-Blackwell.

Muggenthaler, M., Singh, A. and Wilkinson, P. (2008) The role of coronary artery stents in PCI. *British Journal of Cardiac Nursing*, **3**(1): 24–30.

National Institute for Health and Care Excellence (NICE) (2013) Myocardial infarction with ST-segment elevation: the acute management of myocardial infarction with ST-segment elevation. *NICE Clinical Guideline 167*.

National Institute for Health and Clinical Excellence (NICE) (2008) Drug-eluting stents for the treatment of coronary artery disease. *NICE Technology Appraisal Guidance*: 152.

National Institute for Health and Clinical Excellence (NICE) (2010a) Unstable angina and NSTEMI: the early management of unstable angina and non-ST-segment-elevation myocardial infarction. *NICE Clinical Guidelines 94.*

National Institute for Health and Clinical Excellence (NICE) (2010b) Chest pain of recent onset: assessment and diagnosis of recent onset chest pain or discomfort of suspected cardiac origin. *NICE Clinical Guidelines 95.*

Theroux, P., Ouimet, H., McCans, J., Latour, J.G., Joly, P., Lévy, G., Pelletier, E., Juneau, M., Stasiak, J., deGuise, P. *et al.* (1988) Aspirin, heparin or both to treat acute unstable angina. *New England Journal of Medicine*, **319**: 1105–1011.

Wordsworth, S. (2014) Professional practice and the operating department practitioner, in Abbott, H. and Booth, H. (eds) *Foundations in Operating Department Practice*. London: Open University Press.

Ziakas, A., Gomma, A., McDonald, J., Klinke, P. and Hilton, D. (2007) A comparison of the radial and the femoral approaches in primary or rescue percutaneous coronary intervention for acute myocardial infarction in the elderly. *Acute Cardiac Care*, **9**(2): 93–96.

Laparoscopic adjustable gastric band: the care of Chloe Brown

Hannah Abbott

INTRODUCTION AND LEARNING OUTCOMES

Obesity is an increasing public health concern in the UK and can be a precursor to a number of other co-morbidities. There are a number of different initiatives to raise awareness of the health implications of obesity and how individuals can address this; these include online advice programmes by the National Health Service (NHS) – for example, the Change4Life initiative – and slimming club membership on prescription. When non-surgical weight loss methods have been exhausted, however, bariatric surgery is recommended for adults with a body mass index (BMI) of 40 or above as this is more effective in achieving and maintaining weight loss; consequently the number of NHS bariatric procedures has increased from approximately 470 in 2003/4 to more than 6500 in 2009/10 (Dent et al., 2010). Bariatric surgery is an umbrella term that encompasses a number of surgical interventions – for example, gastric banding, Roux-en-Y gastric bypass and sleeve gastrectomy. The aim of bariatric surgery is to achieve weight loss through reducing the stomach volume, which results in satiety after small volumes of food.

This case study explores the perioperative journey of a female patient undergoing a laparoscopic adjustable gastric band procedure.

By the end of this case study you will be able to:

- explain the indications for bariatric surgery and the preparation of the patient
- discuss the intraoperative care of the patient
- consider the immediate and long-term postoperative care of the patient
- discuss the wider care considerations for the patient.

Case outline

Chloe Brown is a 17-year-old female who presents as morbidly obese at 5 ft 5 in tall and 112 kg, giving her a BMI of 41. Chloe has always been overweight as a teenager and weighed 15 stone (95.3 kg) when she turned 15, however her weight has increased over the past two years due to changes in her

---

circumstances, which have resulted in a poor diet and comfort eating. Chloe previously lived with her mother and stepfather, where her diet consisted of large portions of convenience foods, however following Chloe's disclosure that she had been sexually abused by her stepfather, she now lives with her biological father. Chloe's father works long hours and so Chloe cooks for herself every evening, often stopping at a takeaway on her way home from sixth form. While Chloe has some friends she often avoids seeing them outside sixth form because they typically want to go clothes shopping, which isolates Chloe as their preferred shops do not cater for her; alternatively they enjoy nights out and socialising (usually with groups of young single men), and Chloe currently finds male attention threatening and uncomfortable. Consequently Chloe spends increasing amounts of time at home, watching TV or studying for her A-levels while comfort eating – mainly chocolate and ice cream.

Chloe feels that her weight is destroying her confidence, which is having an adverse effect on her emotional well-being and career aspirations; she would like to become a primary school teacher, however she feels that she lacks the confidence to stand in front of a class or even to attend a university interview. Chloe has made attempts to lose weight on her own and has tried a range of approaches, including intermittent fasting, a high-protein diet and a meal-replacement diet, in addition to attempting two different regimes prescribed by her general practitioner (GP), a weight loss group and, subsequently, appetite-suppressing drugs. She has not however been able to sustain any of these and after a period of initial weight loss returns to her current eating habits. She has also attempted to exercise but feels too large and uncomfortable and, following some recent unpleasant comments when attempting to go for a run, has ceased any attempt at increasing her physical activity. This experience is not uncommon, as it has been recognised that successful weight loss using diet and exercise alone is unusual in patients with a BMI exceeding 40 (Zitsman, 2014).

Chloe feels that the only remaining weight loss option is surgical intervention; she has discussed this with her father and GP. Chloe does not fully meet the criteria for bariatric surgery as, while her BMI exceeds 40, she has exhausted appropriate non-surgical measures, has committed to the requirement for long-term follow-up and is generally fit and well, she has not yet received intensive management in a Tier 3 service (NICE, 2014). It was therefore decided that Chloe should first fully engage with Tier 3 services and she was referred to a community care multidisciplinary team (MDT) that could provide 'an intense level of input' (NHS Commissioning Board, 2013: 7) to try alternative non-surgical interventions.

While Chloe is currently generally fit and well, Zitsman (2014) believes that obesity at a young age is likely to continue into adulthood with the associated risk of obesity-related complications – for example, type 2 diabetes, hypertension and obstructive sleep apnoea. Despite this, however, NICE (2014) does not advocate bariatric surgery for young people, unless in exceptional circumstances when they are close to physiological maturity. Early trials in the United

States, however, have suggested that laparoscopic adjustable gastric banding (LAGB) is an effective weight loss technique in adolescents, whose results are comparable with those for adults (Zitsman, 2014) and, given Chloe's medical history and physiological maturity, she is supported in her desire to arrange a private referral to a bariatric surgeon.

Following further discussion with her father and the bariatric surgeon, Chloe decides to proceed with bariatric surgery privately, which is funded by her father and is scheduled at the beginning of the summer holidays to allow Chloe to have maximum time to recover before returning to sixth form. The consultant explained the range of bariatric surgical procedures and, following discussion, it was agreed that LAGB would be best suited to her as, while the weight loss is at a slower rate than with gastric bypass, it is fully reversible and is the safest and quickest option, with a low incidence of major perioperative complications (Kerrigan, Magee and Mitchell, 2011).

Stop and think

Before reading further, think about the patient who is presenting for surgery. What care does she require? You should consider her physical care needs, in particular the impact of obesity upon her care. You should also consider the procedural requirements and how these may impact upon other areas of her care – for example, the anaesthetic technique. It is essential however that you also consider her psychological care needs, as well as the impact of her personal and social history upon her perioperative care and recovery.

First, consider the preoperative stage of Chloe's care, as this is an essential component of her perioperative care.

1   **What physical assessments are essential and must be undertaken for Chloe, considering her morbid obesity?**

A   Chloe attends the pre-assessment clinic two weeks prior to her scheduled surgery, where a full preoperative assessment is undertaken, including an assessment by her anaesthetist. The anaesthetic assessment considers specifically the areas that present specific risks to patients who are obese. Chloe's airway was assessed, she had a Mallampati score of 2 and class II upper lip bite test, neither of which suggest difficult intubation; due to her obesity however she has fat accumulation in the tissue of the neck, which restricts her head and neck extension and this, in addition to a positive submental sign, could indicate difficult intubation. Due to her obesity, Chloe has a reduced functional residual capacity (FRC), which will result in an increased rate of desaturation in the event of a difficult intubation (AAGBI, 2007); the team will therefore be prepared for any potential difficulty in intubation and can position the patient to improve visualisation during laryngoscopy by raising the patient's head, upper body and shoulders above the chest (Sabharwal and Christelis, 2010). Chloe

is assessed for any respiratory co-morbidities, which are common in morbid obesity –
for example, sleep apnoea or wheezing – and also for any co-existing respiratory
co-morbidities – for example, asthma (AAGBI, 2007); however Chloe does not present
with any of these. Chloe is assessed for signs of cardiac disease and metabolic
disease, as these are common in obese patients (AAGBI, 2007), however she does
not present with any of these.

2   **Before bariatric surgery Chloe must follow a specific preoperative diet. What does
this involve and what is the physiological reason for this?**

A   At pre-assessment Chloe is given a preoperative diet sheet that she must adhere to
rigidly for the two weeks until her surgery. This is a low-calorie diet that is low in
carbohydrates and low in fat. The diet is designed to reduce the glycogen stores in
the body, especially those in the liver, thus reducing the overall size of the liver,
which will aid surgical access to the stomach. In addition to following the diet plan,
Chloe is advised to take some exercise every day according to her own physical
ability.

3   **On the day of admission, what preoperative assessments and preparations are
required for Chloe? Try to consider the mitigation of risks associated with caring for
morbidly obese patients.**

A   Chloe is admitted on the morning of her surgery having fasted at home in accordance
with the preoperative fasting guidelines. Routine observations are recorded on admission and Chloe is administered metoclopramide (10 mg) and oral ranitidine (150 mg);
this is a prophylactic measure for aspiration and is considered good practice for all
patients even if they do not report a history of reflux (Sabharwal and Christelis,
2010). Obese patients present a significant risk of venous thromboembolism with DVT
being the most frequent postoperative complication of bariatric surgery (Sabharwal
and Christelis, 2010) and therefore Chloe is fitted with graduated compression stockings; it is essential that there are a range of sizes for both width and length as Chloe
is 5 ft 5 in tall, and so requires relatively short knee-length stockings that are of a
sufficient calf circumference.

4   **The perioperative team must prepare the theatre environment prior to surgery.
What specific checks must be undertaken to ensure the safe care of Chloe as a
morbidly obese patient?**

A   The specific preparation of the theatre environment for bariatric surgery is primarily
to manage the obese patient and it is therefore important for the theatre team to
have information regarding the weight (in kilograms) of the patient. The team must
ensure that there are sufficient team members to move Chloe, although a weight of
112 kg is unlikely to require additional staff for manual handling. The team however
prepare a hover mattress to assist with the lateral transfer; this is placed under Chloe
and, once inflated, becomes an air cushion that supports the patient. On the under-
side there are small holes that allow the air to escape, which reduces friction on the
transfer, allowing the team to 'glide' Chloe from her bed to the operating table. The
weight limit of the operating table must be checked to ensure it is sufficient; it is also
likely that side extenders will be required to increase the width of the table; these are

typically placed in the abdominal area, which is appropriate for Chloe as this is where she has a high proportion of excess fat. Footplates are also attached to the table as Chloe will be placed in a steep reverse Trendelenburg position and the footplates prevent the patient sliding.

Chloe's obesity is considered when preparing all the different equipment for use. For example, she will require a large blood pressure cuff and large intermittent calf compressors. It is important that a range of appropriate sizes are prepared in advance as it would be embarrassing for Chloe if delays were caused by members of the theatre team having to leave to find larger-sized equipment. It is also important that sufficient members of the team are available to safely undertake manual handling tasks as required to ensure the safety of Chloe and the team.

Now consider Chloe's anaesthetic care both in the context of her morbid obesity and the procedure she is having

5 **What anaesthetic technique do you think is most appropriate, and why? How can this be delivered safely at both induction and emergence?**

A Chloe will undergo her surgery under general anaesthesia with endotracheal intubation as there is a risk of regurgitation and aspiration. Prior to induction, routine observations are recorded; as Chloe did not have any co-morbidities, additional invasive monitoring was not considered necessary. Pre-oxygenation is essential prior to induction and Chloe is asked to breathe oxygen via a face mask; this results in the denitrogenation of the FRC, which increases tolerance to apnoea and therefore is particularly pertinent in Chloe's case, where there is potential for difficult intubation. Chloe has no history of reflux and is adequately fasted, therefore the anaesthetist does not consider that a rapid sequence induction (RSI) is required in her case; a number of obese patients do experience reflux and so an RSI may be required prior to bariatric surgery. Propofol is used for induction, along with the non-depolarising muscle relaxant atracurium, and a remifentanil infusion is commenced. Chloe was intubated with the aid of a bougie and the cuffed endotracheal tube was secured. An oral gastric tube was also inserted and will be used during surgery to decompress the stomach (Sabharwal and Christelis, 2010). Chloe also has prophylactic antibiotics and a remifentanil infusion as her intraoperative analgesic, as this can be easily titrated according to the clinical need. At the end of the procedure, and following adequate reversal, Chloe was extubated on her bed in a semi-sitting position (Blanshard, 2011) and then transferred to the post-anaesthetic care unit (PACU).

6 **What other measures will be undertaken to maintain homeostasis?**

A Chloe is administered intravenous crystalloid fluid, via a fluid warmer, throughout her surgery, with the rate of administration adjusted according to clinical need. In accordance with NICE (2008) guidelines, a forced air warming device was applied and used from induction of anaesthesia. Chloe's temperature was also monitored and recorded at 30-minute intervals throughout the procedure.

Evidence-based care: pharmacology of anaesthetic agents in the obese patient

Some studies have explored the impact of obesity upon the clinical pharmacology of anaesthetic drugs, however although obese patients have an increased lean body mass of 20–40%, there is also a greater increase of fat mass per kilogram of total body weight, which results in an overall decrease in lean body mass per kilogram of body weight; these changes affect the apparent volume of distribution in obese patients (Ingrande, Brodsky and Lemmens, 2011). These physiological changes must be considered when selecting the appropriate drug regime for the patient. As a hydrophilic drug, atracurium has a similar volume of distribution in obese and non-obese patients, hence the dose is calculated by lean body mass; there is also no significant difference in recovery time (Sabharwal and Christelis, 2010; Blanshard, 2011). By contrast, propofol is lipophilic and has a high volume of distribution, which was considered when calculating the appropriate induction dose. The high proportion of body fat in obese patients is thought to act as a reservoir for volatile maintenance agents; this is believed to delay emergence and may contribute to residual airway obstruction (Vallejo *et al.*, 2007). Consequently Sabhaewal and Christelis (2010) advocate the use of desflurane due to the low blood:gas partition coefficient, which they believe results in an improved recovery profile. The randomised controlled trial by Vallejo *et al.* (2007) has shown comparable recovery characteristics for sevoflurane and desflurane in morbidly obese patients; there was no significant difference in length of stay in the PACU between groups (P=0.08), although the mean stay of the desflurane group (160.2 minutes) was longer than that for the sevoflurane group (144.3 minutes); the nausea scores however were significantly higher (P=0.03) in the desflurane group than in the sevoflurane group.

Now think about the surgical approach for this surgery

7   What does the surgical technique involve?

A   Once skin preparation and draping has been completed to prepare the sterile field, the surgery commences with the insertion of the laparoscopic port sites. Once the first port is inserted, the insufflation gas (carbon dioxide) begins to inflate the abdominal cavity and the remaining ports are inserted; in total there are five ports of which four are 5 mm and one is 15 mm. In order to expose the oesophagogastric area, a Nathanson liver retractor is inserted via a small incision; this is specifically designed for retraction of the liver – it evenly distributes the weight of the liver and is fixed in position with the appropriate table attachment (Zitsman, 2014).

A retrogastric tunnel is created via blunt dissection, and a standard-sized gastric band inserted via the 15 mm port. This tubing was threaded through the retrogastric tunnel before connecting back to the band and securing it in place so that the band sits just below the gastro-oesophageal junction and creates a small gastric pouch (Beitner and Kurian, 2012; Zitsman, 2014). The band is typically sutured into place between the fundus and gastric pouch with a non-absorbable suture, as this is believed to reduce complications related to the band slipping (Kerrigan et al., 2011); Zitsman (2014), however, questions the efficacy of this suturing approach and suggests fixation of the stomach to the left upper port site, although at present there does not appear to be any empirical evidence to support the efficacy of this technique. The inflation tubing is then connected to the injection port, which is inserted subcutaneously and attached to the rectus sheath fascia (Beitner and Kurian, 2012).

8 **What is the rationale for the decisions related to closure of the port site incisions and what are the risks associated with this?**

A Once the ports and Nathanson retractor have been removed, the fascia at the 15 mm port site is closed with sutures; this is to minimise the risk of complications at the port site, such as herniation. The 5 mm port sites are closed with skin glue as it is not considered necessary to close the fascia level for sites from ports less than 10 mm, although it is still possible for an incisional hernia to occur at these sites (Botea, Torzilli and Sarbu, 2011). All the sites were dressed with small, permeable self-adhesive dressings prior to the removal of the surgical drapes.

9 **How was the most appropriate location for Chloe's postoperative care determined?**

A The most appropriate location for a patient's immediate post-anaesthetic care following bariatric surgery can be determined by calculating their Montefiore Obesity Surgery Score (MOSS). As Chloe was under 50 years old, with no history of asthma or snoring, it was appropriate to care for her in the PACU (Sabharwal and Christelis, 2010). Chloe will have the same full assessment as all patients in the post-anaesthetic care unit (PACU), however there are some specific considerations for her.

10 **Chloe had specifically asked for a female practitioner to care for her in the PACU. Why do you think this may be?**

A Chloe was assigned a female PACU practitioner; this was at Chloe's request as she was concerned that it would be distressing for her to awake to find a male standing over her. While Chloe knew she was in a safe place, she disclosed that she had distressing nightmares following a period of sexual abuse, and was concerned that when confused and disorientated from the anaesthetic, she would panic to find a male in close proximity as she awoke.

11 **Maintaining adequate oxygenation is essential for all patients postoperatively. How do you think this can be optimised in Chloe's case? (You should consider her BMI.)**

A Chloe had been extubated in theatre and was transferred to the PACU with oxygen via a venturi mask as these ensure that a fixed concentration of oxygen can be delivered and prevent rebreathing. It has been suggested that commencing postoperative incentive spirometry or continuous positive airway pressure (CPAP) in the PACU is beneficial in improving the return of preoperative pulmonary function (Sabharwal and Christelis, 2010), although this was not felt to be necessary for Chloe. Chloe was however positioned in a semi-seated position in her bed, with the back rest at approximately 45°. It is beneficial if the patient is in an electrically controlled bed as this allows easy adjustment of their position without increasing the manual handling for staff. Chloe was monitored with routine PACU monitoring as detailed in the Introduction.

12 **Control of pain is a key element of PACU care. What do you think the appropriate assessment and management of pain would be for Chloe?**

A Effective pain assessment and management is important following bariatric surgery as it maximises ventilation (as the patient is not in pain when taking deep breaths), thus reducing the risk of postoperative chest infection. Chloe had received local anaesthetic infiltration to the port sites in theatre and had patient-controlled anaesthesia (PCA) prescribed for the PACU; this is usually sufficient for laparoscopic procedures (Sabharwal and Christelis, 2010). Chloe's pain was assessed using the numerical rating scale, which is simple to use and allows differentiation between different levels of pain (Abbott, 2014); Chloe reported a pain score of 5 for abdominal pain, but also reported referred pain in her shoulders as a result of the insufflation gas, and was encouraged to use her PCA accordingly. When Chloe had met the recovery discharge criteria of stable observations, controlled pain and emesis, she was discharged back to the ward to continue her recovery.

Finally, consider the longer-term postoperative care and support, as this is essential for Chloe to achieve the weight loss she requires.

13 **Why was Chloe encouraged to mobilise as soon as possible after surgery?**

A Due to the increased risk of thromboembolism Chloe was advised to mobilise as soon as possible following her return to the ward, and to continue to do so throughout her recovery. While LAGB can be performed as a day case, this was not usual practice in this hospital and so Chloe was discharged the next day with follow-up appointments arranged. Day surgery however does offer a number of advantages for obese patients and one of these is prompt mobilisation, therefore it is important that Chloe mobilises on the ward and is aware of the importance of this.

14 **When will Chloe be able to eat and drink again, and how will this progress to a full range of foods?**

A Immediately after her surgery Chloe's intake is restricted to fluids only and, after day two, this is increased to a liquid diet. Over the next few weeks Chloe follows the hospital postoperative diet regime, progressing from puréed food to a soft diet, and finally being able to eat normally after approximately four weeks. She is however given advice that some foods' textures may be more difficult for her and can block the band, so she has been advised to avoid these. She must also eat slowly and chew her food well. Chloe therefore has to learn to eat in a different way and must also avoid drinking with meals and fizzy drinks, however her father has taken some time off work and she finds that eating at the dining table with him helps her to eat more slowly and deliberately than when she was eating alone watching TV.

15 **What ongoing postoperative care is required for Chloe? (You should consider nutritional advice and psychological support.)**

A The aim of the LAGB is that Chloe will lose between 1 and 2 lb (0.45–0.91 kg (2 dp)) per week; she will be reviewed by her consultant and dietician regularly after surgery to monitor her progress. At these appointments the band will be reviewed and may be adjusted if necessary. If this is required, fluid will be injected into or removed from the band via the subcutaneous port site according to the adjustment required.

Chloe was given ongoing nutritional advice and is advised to attend a bariatric surgery support group as, unlike gastric bypass, the success of her weight loss will depend upon her motivation to follow the nutritional advice. This is particularly import-ant to Chloe, who is a comfort eater and favours chocolate and ice cream, which can still be consumed post-banding; therefore failure to significantly reduce her intake of these will adversely affect her weight loss By contrast, had Chloe undergone gastric bypass she would have experienced 'dumping' syndrome following the consumption of sugary carbohydrates (Kerrigan *et al.*, 2011). Chloe is aware that her comfort eat-ing is partially due to her low self-esteem as a result of her obesity and partially resulting from the distress caused by her stepfather's abuse and her mother's sub-sequent rejection of her. Consequently she opts to attend counselling to address these issues.

16 **Why is Chloe given contraceptive advice after her surgery?**

A The general consensus is that patients should delay pregnancy until 12–18 months post-surgery as this allows sufficient time to adapt to the gastric band, to maximise weight loss and to reduce potential complications relating to nutritional deficiencies (Kominiarek, 2011). There is limited evidence to suggest differences in perinatal outcomes early after bariatric surgery, however a matched cohort study has sug-gested that there is an increased risk of small-for-gestational-age infants ($P<0.001$), and possibly reduced gestation and increased risk of neonatal death (Johansson *et al.*, 2015).

Chloe should receive information regarding contraception and future pregnancy, although she has no current desire for a relationship. Should Chloe become pregnant in the future she will be managed in consultation with the bariatric team as there are different approaches to management, with some advocating deflation of the band to reduce the risk of complications – for example, band migration or nausea and vomiting. Alternatively, in other cases, the band may be adjusted only if the patient fails to gain weight in pregnancy or experiences vomiting (Kominiarek, 2011).

17 **What is the long-term aim of the surgery?**

A If Chloe adheres to the nutritional advice following her surgery she can expect to lose 1 to 2 lb (0.45–0.91 kg (2 dp)) per week and approximately 50% of her excess weight within two years. This should therefore reduce her risk of developing obesity-related co-morbidities in the future.

REFERENCES AND FURTHER READING

Abbott, H. (2014) Perioperative assessment, in Abbott, H., Braithwaite, W. and Ranson, M. (eds) *Clinical Examination Skills for Healthcare Professionals*. Keswick: M&K Publishing.

Association of Anaesthetists of Great Britain and Ireland (AAGBI) (2007) *Peri-operative Management of the Morbidly Obese Patient*. London: AAGBI.

Beitner, M. and Kurian, M.S. (2012) Laparoscopic adjustable gastric banding. *Abdominal Imaging*, **37**: 687–690.

Blanshard, H. (2011) Endocrine and metabolic disease, in Allman, K.G. and Wilson, I.H. (eds) *Oxford Handbook of Anaesthesia* (3rd edn). Oxford: Oxford University Press.

Botea, F., Torzilli, G. and Sarbu, V. (2011) A simple, effective technique for port-site closure after laparoscopy. *Journal of the Society of Laparoendoscopic Surgeons*, **15**(1): 77–80.

Dent, M., Chrisopoulos, S., Mulhall, C. and Ridler, C. (2010) *Bariatric Surgery for Obesity*. Oxford: National Obesity Observatory.

Ingrande, J., Brodsky, J.B. and Lemmens, H.J.M. (2011) Lean body weight scalar for the anesthetic induction dose of propofol in morbidly obese subjects. *Anesthesia and Analgesia*, **113**(1): 57–62.

Johansson, K., Cnattingius, S., Näslund, I., Roos, N., Lagerros, Y.T., Granath, F., Stephansson, O. and Neovius, M. (2015) Outcomes of pregnancy after bariatric surgery. *New England Journal of Medicine*, **372**: 814–824.

Kerrigan, D., Magee, C. and Mitchell, A.I. (2011) Bariatric surgery. *Surgery*, **29**(1): 581–585.

Kominiarek, M.A. (2011) Preparing for and managing a pregnancy after bariatric surgery. *Seminars in Perinatology*, **35**(6): 356–361.

National Institute for Health and Care Excellence (NICE) (2014) Identification, assessment and management of overweight and obesity in children, young people and adults. Partial update of CG43. Available online at: www.nice.org.uk/guidance/cg189/evidence/obesity-update-full-guideline-193342429 (accessed 27 October 2015).

National Institute for Health and Clinical Excellence (NICE) (2008) Inadvertent perioperative hypothermia. *NICE Clinical Guideline 65*. Available online at: www.nice.org.uk/guidance/cg65/resources/guidance-inadvertent-perioperative-hypothermia-pdf (accessed 21 September 2014).

NHS Commissioning Board (2013) Clinical commissioning policy: complex and specialised obesity surgery. Available online at: www.england.nhs.uk/wp-content/uploads/2013/04/a05-p-a.pdf (accessed 19 September 2014).

Sabharwal, A. and Christelis, N. (2010) Anaesthesia for bariatric surgery. *Continuing Education in Anaesthesia*, **10**(4): 99–103.

Vallejo, M.C., Sah, N., Phelps, A.L., O'Donnell, J. and Romeo, R.C. (2007) Desflurane versus sevoflurane for laparoscopic gastroplasty in morbidly obese patients. *Journal of Clinical Anesthesia*, **19**: 3–8.

Zitsman, J.L. (2014) Laparoscopic adjustable gastric banding in adolescents. *Seminars in Pediatric Surgery*, **23**: 17–23.

CASE STUDY 19

Laparoscopic nephrectomy: the care of Pamela Wilkinson

Sue Parker

INTRODUCTION AND LEARNING OUTCOMES

The laparoscopic approach for simple nephrectomy has become the standard for managing patients with permanent loss of renal function caused by benign renal disease (Gupta and Guatman, 2005) and will form the basis of this case study. The National Institute for Health and Clinical Excellence (now the National Institute for Health and Care Excellence) supports the safety and efficacy of laparoscopic nephrectomy (NICE, 2005). Indications for the procedure include: kidney cancer, trauma to kidney and benign disease such as hydronephrosis, chronic infection, polycystic kidney disease, shrunken kidney, hypertension or renal calculus (NICE, 2005). More recent advances in laparoscopic surgical techniques have enabled this procedure to be undertaken effectively as a day case (Ilie *et al.*, 2011).

Although the main focus of this case study is on the laparoscopic approach, it is important to acknowledge that an open approach may sometimes be considered necessary or, if complications arise during laparoscopic surgery such as inability to control excessive bleeding, then the procedure may convert to open.

By the end of this case study you will be able to:

- describe the pre-, peri- and postoperative care of the patient undergoing laparoscopic nephrectomy
- explain the rationale for the use of a laparoscopic approach for nephrectomy
- discuss the day case approach to laparoscopic nephrectomy.

Case outline

Pamela Wilkinson is a 57-year-old female with a history of chronic nephritis, which has resulted in renal failure in the right kidney. Her medical history indicates type 2 diabetes, which is currently diet controlled, two previous Caesarean sections and a total abdominal hysterectomy five years ago for fibroids. She has no known drug allergies. According to her notes and pre-admission assessment she was a previous grade 2 intubation.

The intention is to perform the surgery as day surgery, the protocol for which has been discussed with the patient in clinic with the consultant urologist. The most important criterion is Mrs Wilkinson's willingness to undergo her operation as day surgery, which includes the following aspects: that she has adequate support in the immediate 24 hours post-surgery by a responsible adult or carer (in this case her husband who has taken three days off work to look after her); access to a telephone to contact the hospital for help and advice; the homeward journey post-discharge should be less than one hour; and that she should be accompanied by a suitable escort (Ilie *et al.*, 2011). She has arranged for her daughter to take her home from the hospital later that afternoon and to wait with her until Mrs Wilkinson's husband finishes work.

Mrs Wilkinson was advised of the risks/benefits and complications associated with this type of surgical intervention, and laparoscopic procedures in particular, in the outpatients clinic in order for her to make an informed decision regarding her treatment. The advantages of a laparoscopic approach over open surgery include no large incision, reduced postoperative pain, shorter hospital stay, earlier return to work and better cosmetic results. There are, however, a number of complications, including bleeding, infection, tissue/organ damage, hernia formation and conversion to open surgery (Bishoff and Kavoussi, 2007).

Stop and think

What are your initial thoughts regarding Mrs Wilkinson's care and the interventions she may require? What do you think her main concerns may be?

1 **What preoperative preparation will be undertaken when Mrs Wilkinson is admitted to the day surgery ward?**

A Mrs Wilkinson was admitted on to a day surgery ward from 7 am for the morning operating list. She has been advised in her admission letter to not have breakfast, but could have clear fluids up to two hours preoperatively. Mrs Wilkinson was listed first on the operating list due to her diabetic status.

The admission process on the day surgery unit comprises taking a brief history from Mrs Wilkinson, which covers her past medical and surgical history, current medication and taking baseline physiological observations. As part of this Mrs Wilkinson was asked her preferred name and expressed that she would prefer to be called 'Mrs Wilkinson' rather than by her first name.

Her physiological observations on admission are documented in her day case admission chart and offer a baseline set of criteria for comparative purposes throughout the perioperative journey.

Mrs Wilkinson's preoperative physiological observations were:

- blood pressure 159/86 mmHg
- heart rate 78 bpm

- oxygen saturation 97%
- temperature 36.3°C
- blood glucose 6.7 mmol.

Stop and think

Look at Mrs Wilkinson's observations. What do these mean to you?
Are they within normal ranges or is there anything that concerns you?

A blood sample was taken and sent for full blood count (FBC) and urea and electrolytes (UE), as well as group and save in case of any occurrence of excessive bleeding during the procedure.

Mrs Wilkinson was changed into a theatre gown, anti-thromboembolus stockings applied, her wedding ring was taped and her two crowns were documented in her notes. She was then seen by both the operating surgeon and anaesthetist, and consented to surgery. The site of the operation (right side) was marked by the surgeon with reference to notes, scans and x-rays. A premedication of 1600 mg slow-release ibuprofen was prescribed by the consultant anaesthetist and administered by the ward nurse. This particular medication is a slow-release non-steroidal anti-inflammatory (NSAID), which provides relief for mild to moderate pain for up to 24 hours, and thus contributes to managing the patient's postoperative pain relief.

An important aspect of the admission process is planning Mrs Wilkinson's discharge, taking into account the patient's social circumstances and involvement of external services such as district nurse and general practitioner (GP) (Wicker, 2010), as well as forming part of the day case criteria discussed earlier (Ilie *et al.*, 2011). Her husband has brought her into hospital and arrangements have been made for her daughter to drive her home after discharge, which was preliminarily arranged for late afternoon/early evening.

2 **How would you and the team ensure that the theatre environment and the team are prepared for Mrs Wilkinson's surgery?**

A All equipment is cleaned and checked prior to use and, in the case of anaesthetic machines, signed for by the anaesthetic practitioner. Operating table, lights and diathermy undergo a pre-use check. Positioning aids, such as back supports and arm retainers, are available. Instruments and sundries are prepared and checked by the surgical practitioner for sterility and accuracy of date.

A team brief is undertaken, with all members of the theatre team present, in accordance with the 5 Steps to Safer Surgery, to discuss the requirements of the operating list and any additional specific information shared relating to the procedures. Because of the patient's previous surgical history of Caesarean sections and hysterectomy, a hand port was considered appropriate as prior abdominal surgery can result in adhesion formation, which may pose technical difficulties during insufflation, trocar placement and dissection (Gupta and Gautman, 2005). The anaesthetist informed the team of the patient's previous intubation grade, which pre-empted the possibility of a difficult intubation and potential equipment required.

3   **How will the patient be prepared for anaesthesia?**

A   Following handover from the ward nurse to the anaesthetic practitioner in the anaesthetic room, which includes accurate identification of the patient, confirmation of written consent for the procedure and completion of stage 1 of the WHO Surgical Safety Checklist, monitoring is applied to Mrs Wilkinson in accordance with minimal monitoring standards (AAGBI, 2007). Due to the positioning of the patient during surgery the blood pressure cuff (NIBP) and pulse oximeter probe are attached to the same arm as the operation side (i.e. uppermost to reduce the risk of inaccurate readings and additional pressure to the arm if the patient were to be lying on it). An intravenous cannula (18G or greater) is also sited on the same uppermost arm and adequately secured. A non-return valve is attached to the giving set to prevent backflow when the blood pressure cycles.

4   **What anaesthetic technique do you think would be most appropriate for this patient and procedure, and why?**

A   Anaesthetic of choice for this surgical procedure is general anaesthesia due to the duration of the procedure being two to three hours, patient position and the use of pneumoperitoneum. The anaesthetic implications associated with laparoscopic procedures relate primarily to production of a pneumoperitoneum and the increase in intra-abdominal pressure. These include bradycardia through vagal nerve stimulation of the peritoneum or occlusion of the inferior vena cava and/or abdominal aorta. Increased pressure on the diaphragm can also contribute to bradycardia. The length of procedure and use of continuous pneumoperitoneum results in the absorption of carbon dioxide, which in turn increases both the amount to be excreted and the respiratory drive. Tracheal intubation and the use of intermittent positive pressure ventilation (IPPV) are thus considered necessary for this procedure (Aitkenhead et al., 2013).

5   **Which drugs and fluids do you think will be used for this case?**

A   In accordance with NICE Guidelines on Inadvertent Hypothermia (NICE, 2008), warmed fluids (compound sodium lactate 1000 ml) were attached to the cannula for intraoperative fluid maintenance. For day case laparoscopic nephrectomy it is advised that the patient receives only 2 litres of fluid intraoperatively. This reduces the need to catheterise the patient and encourages postoperative micturition, which is an indicator for discharge. It further reduces overfilling of the bladder, which may lead to urinary retention.

The drugs used for Mrs Wilkinson, and their rationale, are listed in Table 19.1.

Towards the end of the surgery, 50 mcg fentanyl and paracetamol (1 g) will be administered intravenously to help with the immediate reversal and recovery process, as well as longer management of postoperative pain relief. At the end of the procedure, reversal of the muscle relaxant will be facilitated through the administration of neostigmine and glycopyrrolate.

Table 19.1 Drugs used in day case laparoscopic nephrectomy

Pre-medication	1600 mg slow-release ibuprofen	Pain relief
Induction	midazolam 2 mg	Sedative used to help alleviate anxiety
	alfentanil 1 mg	Short-acting analgesic, aids in induction process and facilitates intubation
	propofol 150 mg	Induction agent that induces anaesthesia with associated benefits of ease of recovery and fewer side effects of PONV
Antibiotic	co-amoxyclav 1.2 mg	Prophylactic antibiotic used to cover invasive procedures
Muscle relaxant	rocuronium	Long-acting muscle relaxant used to facilitate intubation and relaxation of muscles to aid surgical process
Anti-emetics	dexamethasone 8 mg ondansetron	Prevents PONV, which is a common associated complication of laparoscopic surgery
Maintenance	sevoflurane	Used to maintain anaesthesia during surgery
Perioperative analgesia	intravenous paracetamol 1 g 50 mcg fentanyl	Helps with immediate and postoperative pain relief
Local analgesia (port site infiltration)	levobupivacaine 0.5% up to 30 ml	Postoperative pain relief

6   **How would Mrs Wilkinson's airway be established?**

A   Once anaesthetised the anaesthetist undertook laryngoscopy to assess Mrs Wilkinson's airway, taking into consideration her past anaesthetic history of being a grade II intubation. Intubation was facilitated using a size 3 Macintosh laryngoscope blade and slight laryngeal pressure to manipulate the larynx into view; a bougie was inserted through the vocal cords and a size 7.0 endotracheal tube railroaded over it. Once placement of the ET tube was established through observation of expired carbon dioxide on the capnograph it was secured using a tie. Mrs Wilkinson's eyes were covered and padded to protect her corneas, and an orogastric tube was inserted to decompress the stomach during surgery.

7   **How was would you position Mrs Wilkinson for her surgery and what do you need to consider when doing this?**

A   Positioning of the patient for the procedure of laparoscopic nephrectomy requires careful planning and cooperation between all members of the theatre team. Mrs Wilkinson is to undergo a right nephrectomy, and is therefore positioned in the left lateral position and angled slightly backwards in a 'flank' position. This position is considered more ergonomic for the patient and optimum for surgical access, in particular for the number and placement of the laparoscopic ports.

Her lower (left) arm was positioned on or under the pillow adjacent to her face. The uppermost arm (right), with monitoring and intravenous cannula in situ, can either be secured in a Carter–Bain arm retainer or placed alongside the lower arm by the side of the patient's head in a natural 'foetal' position. Care was taken not to incur any pressure on her face and also to ensure that her arms and hands were both adequately supported and secure from being displaced. Alternatively, an arm board may be used to support both arms, with adequate padding such as blankets or pillows between them in order to reduce the risk of pressure area development. If specific pressure-relieving aids are available these should be used where possible. Care should be taken to ensure all intravenous lines and patient monitoring leads are not trapped under the patient as these may cause pressure area necrosis from the weight of the patient.

The patient was secured in the lateral position through the use of Elastoplast over her hip and shoulder to anchor her to the table; back and abdominal supports may be used as an alternative. The use of strapping reduces the impingement of the table supports on the surgeon's accessibility while undertaking the procedure. If table straps are being used, ensure that padding is placed between the straps and the patient. Mrs Wilkinson's lower leg was flexed at the knee and hip, and her upper leg remained extended. Special attention was paid to the padding of any pressure points. A pillow or pillows were placed between her legs to reduce pressure and nerve damage, particularly around the knee and ankle. Pillows were used due to their lightness in comparison with some specifically designed pressure-relieving aids, which may increase the weight on to the lower limb. This helps in supporting the upper leg and maintaining patient stability during the procedure. While it was important that Mrs Wilkinson was anchored very securely, care was taken not to anchor her too tightly around the thorax as over-compression of this area may result in an increase in her inspiratory airway pressures.

After being placed in the desired 'flank' position, the table was 'broken' to optimise the surgeon's working space. Over-flexing of the operating table should be avoided, especially in very lean patients, as this may limit the expansion of the abdominal wall and thus reduce the working space available during the procedure.

8 **What other interventions are necessary during surgery? (You should consider the maintenance of homeostasis and the patient monitoring required.)**

A Patient warming (forced air warming) was applied once positioned: a surgical access 'Bair Hugger' was used in this instance; alternatively, an upper and lower body blanket (depending on which is readily available within your particular department) could work as well. It was important to ensure that the operation site was sufficiently exposed for surgical access, but of equal importance was coverage of Mrs Wilkinson's body to help reduce any incurrence of inadvertent hypothermia. The warming device was not turned on until the access ports had been inserted as the inflated blanket(s) can be in the surgeon's way during port insertion. Mrs Wilkinson's temperature was monitored using an oral temperature probe, which was inserted at intubation and secured to the endotracheal tube. A tympanic thermometer could be used as an alternative. The use of an oral temperature probe, although invasive, can be beneficial in providing continuous measurements during a long procedure, whereas the tympanic is less invasive but, due to limited access to the patient during surgery, can be difficult to take, and requires regular and repeated measurement. Intermittent compression devices were attached to the patient's legs to reduce the risk of deep vein thrombosis (DVT).

Mrs Wilkinson's vital signs were measured throughout the procedure and accurately documented on an anaesthetic chart. Due to her diabetes, her blood glucose levels were taken one hour into the procedure to ensure they were maintained within safe limits. Changes in her physiological status were responded to by the anaesthetist; additional doses of the muscle relaxant rocuronium were administered as the previous dose wore off, and a second litre of Hartmann's solution put up and run through slowly. Mrs Wilkinson displayed signs of hypertension during surgery, which was a response to the compression of the inferior vena cava caused by pneumoperitoneum rather than a response to pain. The anaesthetist responded by increasing the inspired percentage of sevoflurane in order to deepen anaesthesia and thus reduce blood pressure rather than administer additional opiates.

9 **What needs to be considered when preparing the theatre for a laparoscopic procedure?**

A Positioning of the laparoscopic monitoring equipment is vital to the surgical procedure. It is recommended that the monitor and image are in direct line of the surgeon; the height of the operating table enables the surgeon to maintain elbows at his/her side in order to reduce muscle fatigue. The surgeon's assistant/camera holder is often seated due to the upward angle of the telescope once inside the abdomen.

10 **What does the surgical technique for this procedure involve?**

A Mrs Wilkinson's abdomen and the whole of her flank were prepped with povidone–iodine 70% in case of conversion to open surgery. A standard transperitoneal approach was used, with four small incisions made in the abdomen through which the required instruments were inserted. A larger incision was made for the use of a port for the technique of hand-assisted laparoscopic nephrectomy. This particular technique allows the surgeon to place one hand in the abdomen while maintaining pneumoperitoneum. A small incision was made, just large enough for the surgeon to place his hand inside, and an airtight 'sleeve' used to form a seal. Typically, the primary surgeon's non-dominant hand works through the hand-assisted device, and his or her dominant hand is used for fine tissue manipulation with a laparoscopic instrument. It further enables retraction of tissues/organs, offers tactile feedback, and provides additional orientation of the surgery and manual compression of bleeding if required (Santos *et al.*, 2003).

A Veress needle is inserted by the umbilicus, which also forms the first trocar/port insertion for the laparoscope. The abdomen is filled with carbon dioxide to achieve pneumoperitoneum, with a maximum pressure of 15 mmHg. The remaining trocars are inserted under direct vision in order reduce damage to organs/vessels/tissues, and to assess the presence of adhesions. The procedure for surgery is as follows: reflection of the colon; dissection of the ureter; identification of the renal hilum; securing of the renal blood vessels; isolation of the upper pole; retrieval of the kidney (Gupta and Gautman, 2005).

Control of blood loss during laparoscopy is paramount to the success of patient recovery, therefore a range of haemostatic agents and tissue sealants are used routinely, including Harmonic scalpel, LigaSure and Floseal. Failure to maintain haemostasis, or complications resulting from previous surgery such as excessive adhesions, could result in conversion to open surgery. A loin or abdominal incision would usually be made. Blood loss for this procedure was approximately 300 ml.

Local anaesthetic (levobupivacaine 0.5% 30 ml) was injected into the port sites for postop pain relief prior to wound closure. The small surgical wounds made by the port sites were closed in this case with skin glue; the larger wound of the hand port was closed with absorbable sutures: 3/0 Vicryl. All wounds were covered with suitable non-adhesive dressings. Once the towels were removed Mrs Wilkinson was transferred on to her bed and put into a sitting position in readiness for transfer to the post-anaesthetic care unit (PACU).

11   **How would you care for Mrs Wilkinson in the post-anaesthetic care unit?**

A   Mrs Wilkinson was transferred to the PACU by the anaesthetist, accompanied by the anaesthetic practitioner, with full monitoring, still intubated being hand ventilated and on oxygen (15 L/min) administered via a Mapelson C (re-breathe) circuit. Once Mrs Wilkinson was breathing adequately for herself and emerging from anaesthesia she was extubated by the anaesthetist according to recommendations (AAGBI, 2013) and care handed over to the recovery practitioner. A simple face mask was used to deliver 5 L/min of oxygen as prescribed while she was in recovery.

An ABCDE approach to her management in the immediate postoperative period was employed by the recovery practitioner, with minimum observations including (AAGBI, 2013):

- level of consciousness
- airway patency
- respiratory rate
- oxygen saturation
- oxygen administration
- blood pressure
- heart rate and rhythm
- pain and intensity
- PONV
- intravenous infusions
- medications administered
- surgical wound/drainage.

Mrs Wilkinson remained in the PACU for approximately three hours post-surgery before being discharged back to the day surgery ward, having met the set discharge criteria (see box). She experienced a degree of moderate pain for which incremental doses of 20 mcg fentanyl were administered intravenously (maximum 100 mcg).

Prochlorperazine 12.5 mg was given for postoperative nausea and vomiting (PONV). Oxygen was reduced once the patient was comfortable and maintaining adequate saturation levels on air, which was comparable with her admission observations.

Discharge criteria

From a safety perspective the patient must have attained the following criteria before she can be discharged back to the ward (AAGBI, 2013; Hatfield, 2014):

- conscious and oriented
- airway reflexes present
- oxygen saturation levels are satisfactory/consistent with preoperative observations
- oxygen prescribed if appropriate
- heart rate and blood pressure should be stable for at least 30 minutes before discharge (BP >100 mmHg systolic) and approximate to normal preoperative values
- temperature of 36°C or above
- wound sites/drains observed to have no excessive or persistent bleeding
- PONV should be adequately controlled
- pain levels are within acceptable parameters assessed by an appropriate pain-scoring tool
- patient documentation complete and medical notes present.

---

12 **What care will Mrs Wilkinson require when she is back on the ward?**

A Once back on the ward Mrs Wilkinson would undergo routine postoperative observations; she would be encouraged to eat and drink, and pass urine. It was important for her recovery to resume normal food and fluid intake in order to manage her diabetes. An integral part of the discharge criteria, particularly for day surgery procedures, is adequate information regarding care during the first 48 hours post-surgery. An example of the information is found in Table 19.2. Those who are inpatients would be transferred to a long-stay ward. Mrs Wilkinson was discharged late that same afternoon and taken home by her daughter.

Table 19.2 Patient information following laparoscopic nephrectomy

General information	Although the operation was undertaken as a day case procedure it may be several days before you feel well
Medication	Mrs Wilkinson was provided with suitable pain relief to take home and advised to take this regularly:
	ibuprofen 1600 mg slow release paracetamol 1 g four times per day codeine phosphate (30/500) prn (supplementary) ondansetron 4 mg

(Continued)

Table 19.2 (Continued)

District nurse	Mrs Wilkinson was advised that the district nurse would visit her on the evening of her discharge and on the following two days; the district nurse would check the wound sites, manage any dressings as necessary and assess the pain relief
Dressings	The dressing covering the wounds needed to be kept clean and dry until removed by the district nurse after 24–48 hours; if it became wet it was advised that it be removed as this could cause wound infection
Stitches	The ward nurse informed Mrs Wilkinson that the stitches over the larger wound would need to be removed by the district or practice nurse; the smaller wounds were fine as they were secured using skin glue
Constipation	This is a common problem following abdominal surgery, and can cause pain and discomfort. Mrs Wilkinson was advised to eat a high-fibre diet and drink plenty of fluids; laxatives were recommended for short-term use if symptoms persisted
Postoperative advice	Further information given to Mrs Wilkinson related to the following common occurrences associated with laparoscopic surgery: • swelling and bruising around the wound sites • nausea (medication will be prescribed for this) • shoulder tip pain • general wind/indigestion • abdominal pain If these persist or are excessive, or any other problems develop in the postoperative period, Mrs Wilkinson was advised to contact the surgical day unit; she was also given access for up to 48 hours to both the urology ward and the surgical admissions unit via the district nurse/GP
Driving	It is advised that Mrs Wilkinson refrain from driving for approximately two weeks following her surgery as the position of the wounds may prevent her performing emergency manoeuvres and the seat belt may be uncomfortable; this may cause her to be liable in the event of an accident
Work and exercise	Regular exercise can help in rehabilitation but must be introduced gradually and carefully; Mrs Wilkinson was advised that if it hurts, don't do it
Returning to work	Returning to work varies between individuals and the type of work they do. It is sensible to refrain from work for a minimum of two weeks. It was recommended that Mrs Wilkinson consult her GP with regard to the best time for her to return to work

Reproduced and adapted by kind permission of Dr Ian Smith, Consultant Anaesthetist, Day Case Lead, UHNS.

REFERENCES AND FURTHER READING

Aitkenhead, A.R., Moppett, I. and Thompson, J. (2013) *Smith and Aitkenhead's Textbook of Anaesthesia: Expert Consult* (6th edn). Edinburgh: Churchill Livingstone.

Association of Anaesthetists of Great Britain and Ireland (AAGBI) (2007) *Recommendations for Standards of Monitoring During Anaesthesia and Recovery* (4th edn). London: AAGBI.

Association of Anaesthetists of Great Britain and Ireland (AAGBI) (2013) *Immediate Post-anaesthesia Recovery.* London: AAGBI.

Bishoff, J.T. and Kavoussi, L.R. (2007) *Atlas of Laparoscopic Urologic Surgery.* Philadelphia: Saunders.

Gupta, P.N. and Gautman, G. (2005) Laparoscopic nephrectomy for benign non functioning kidneys. *Journal of Minimum Access Surgery*, **1**(4): 149–154.

Hatfield, A. (2014) *The Complete Recovery Room Book* (5th edn). Oxford: Oxford University Press.

Ilie, C.P., Luscombe, C., Smith, I., Boddy, J., Mischianu, D. and Golash, A. (2011) Day case laparoscopic nephrectomy. *Journal of Endourology*, **25**(4): 631–634.

National Institute for Health and Clinical Excellence (NICE) (2005) Laparoscopic nephrectomy (including nephroureterectomy). Available online at: www.nice.org.uk/CGip227overview (accessed 23 April 2014).

National Institute for Health and Clinical Excellence (NICE) (2008) Management of inadvertent perioperative hypothermia in adults. Available online at: www.nice.org.uk/CG065 (accessed 13 May 2014).

Santos, L., Varashin, A.E., Meyer, F., Branco, A., Koleski, F. and Carvalho, R. (2003) Hand-assisted laparoscopic nephrectomy in living donor. *International Brazilian Journal of Urology*, **29**(1): 11–17.

Wicker, P. (2010) Pre-operative preparation of peri-operative patients, in Wicker, P. and O'Neill, J. (eds) *Caring for the Peri-operative Patient.* Chichester: Wiley-Blackwell.

Organ retrieval: the care of Trent Johnston

Ella Davies

INTRODUCTION AND LEARNING OUTCOMES

Organ transplant is an area that is being given more attention in the current climate and so, before beginning this case, having some background knowledge will be beneficial. In the UK an average of three people die each day waiting for an organ transplant. There are currently approximately 7000 people on the active transplant list, and many more die before they even get on to the list. Due to an increase in the ageing population and scientific advances that mean more people are able to benefit from an organ transplant, the number of people needing a transplant is expected to continue to rise. However, the number of organs available for transplant has remained relatively static and the gap between the number of organs donated and the number of people waiting for a transplant is growing. While some types of transplant can be achieved by using organs from living donors, most patients are reliant upon organs from deceased donors. In order to try to reduce the shortfall in the number of donated organs the Department of Health (DH) assembled an Organ Donation Task Force to attempt to identify and resolve some of the obstacles, and increase the number of transplants performed each year in the UK (NHSBT, 2013). The task force concluded that a 50% increase in organ donation was possible within five years provided that some keys issues were resolved. Three of the issues it identified were that there needed to be a method of effective identification and referral of suitable donors, an improvement in donor coordination and management, and efficient organ retrieval arrangements. The task force produced guidance in the form of the National Standards for Organ Retrieval from Deceased Donors; this guidance now provides the framework for a high-quality national organ retrieval service (NORS) in the UK (NHSBT, 2013).

By the end of this case study you will be able to:

- explain the immediate care of the patient on admission to the emergency department
- summarise the principles of donor management
- discuss the effective care and management of a patient prior to, during and after organ donation
- discuss the wider issues related to organ donation and care of the deceased patient in the perioperative environment.

Case outline

Mr Trent Johnston is a 57-year-old male. He has a BMI (body mass index) of 35 and a past medical history of hypertension, which was treated with medication; he has no other relevant medical history and is a non-smoker.

Mr Johnston was admitted into the emergency department (ED) after experiencing what he described at the time as the worst headache he'd ever known, together with a severe vomiting episode while at work. His subsequent collapse was witnessed by his work colleague who, after calling an ambulance, accompanied Mr Johnston to hospital. On admission to ED Mr Johnston had a Glasgow Coma Score (GCS) of 3, indicating no eye opening, no verbal responses and no motor movements. His airway had been secured prior to transfer to hospital by the attending paramedic team using a supra-glottic airway (i-Gel). He had irregular breathing, so this was being supplemented manually via a bag valve mask (BVM). A full trauma team were present in ED on his arrival and an ABCDE assessment was undertaken. The management of his airway was taken over by the on-call anaesthetist and it was very quickly evident that a protected airway needed to be in place. Mr Johnston had recently eaten breakfast and after supplemental breathing with the BVM there was a risk of air being present in the stomach and any stomach contents being aspirated into his lungs. In order to protect his airway, a modified rapid sequence induction was planned; 50 mg of propofol (induction agent) and 100 mcg of suxamethonium (depolarising muscle relaxant) was administered intravenously, full cricoid pressure was used and a cuffed oral endotracheal tube (size 8 with supraglottic suction) was inserted. His breathing was then managed via a portable ventilator, and ongoing sedation and muscle relaxant was administered. He remained hypertensive, hyperthermic and tachycardic, and his pupils were miotic throughout. After the initial assessment and stabilisation a CT scan showed a massive primary pontine haemorrhage with intraventricular extension that was considered unsuitable for surgical intervention. Primary pontine haemorrhages are frequently caused by hypertensive cerebrovascular disease and the haemorrhage usually develops from degenerative arteriolar changes. It carries a poor prognosis and mortality is reported to be between 30% and 68.7% (Wessels *et al.*, 2004).

Stop and think

How much do you understand about intra-cranial haemorrhage? Try to find out some more about this in general and then explore primary pontine haemorrhage. What factors may contribute to this?

1   What does the ongoing management and assessment of Mr Johnston in the intensive care unit involve?

A   Mr Johnston's ongoing management was then taken over by the ICU intensivists and the critical care team on the intensive care unit. As there was no improvement or change in Mr Johnston's clinical status after several days, discussions with the family were undertaken with regard to withdrawal of organ support and possible donation of organs after brain death (DBD). DBD is defined as the retrieval of organs after confirmation of death using brain stem death testing criteria (Cota, Burgess and English, 2013).

   The decision was made that continuing life-sustaining treatment was no longer in Mr Johnston's best interests and should be discontinued. This discussion involved the whole critical care team as well as the family and the known wishes of Mr Johnston. It was at this point that the specialist nurse in organ donation was contacted in order to facilitate the patient optimisation, and subsequent coordination and management of the various retrieval teams and processes. In order for a diagnosis of brain stem death testing the following criteria must be applied:

- the person must be unconscious and fail to respond to outside stimulation
- their breathing can be maintained only using a ventilator
- there must be clear evidence that serious brain damage has occurred and cannot be cured.

Before testing for brain stem death a series of checks are made to ensure that any symptoms aren't being caused by other factors. Once this has been done two senior doctors, not involved with the transplant team, must carry out an independent test to confirm brain stem death. Both doctors have to agree on the result for the confirmation to be made (Smith, 2003).

2   How can consent for organ donation be obtained?

A   Consent for organ retrieval can be obtained by accessing the donor register, although communication with the family and gaining their assent is an important part of the process; it is unlikely that organ donation would go ahead without this. The successful shift in emphasis from a patient-centred approach to a protocol-driven organ management approach must be managed in a sensitive, cohesive manner by the critical care team, the specialist nurse in organ donation, theatre staff and the medical team (NICE, 2011).

3   Now that it has been decided to proceed with organ donation, what management will Mr Johnston require?

A   The basic principles of organ donor management are based on standard treatments and monitoring widely used in ICU throughout the UK, and ICU medical and nursing care is required to optimise the patient and support the relatives. Best supportive care should always be continued in the period between making a decision to withdraw life-sustaining treatment and organ donation. Once this decision has been made and brain stem death has been confirmed, there is usually a shift in the emphasis from active treatment to supportive measures that facilitate organ donation. It is important to ensure, however, that this change in emphasis does not cause harm or distress to the patient (Cota *et al.*, 2013).

A summary of the principles of donor management, as recommended by McKeown, Bonser and Kellum (2012), is as follows.

All unnecessary drugs, including sedatives, should be stopped. A target body temperature of >35°C should be maintained before and during surgery. All active infections should be identified and treated in the lead-up to withdrawal of life-sustaining treatment. Lung-protective ventilation should aim for a tidal volume of 6–8 ml/kg with optimal PEEP to allow for minimum FiO_2 (fractional inspired oxygen). Lung recruitment and chest x-ray should follow any apnoea testing or tracheal suctioning, and the cuff pressure of the endotracheal tube should be maintained at 25 cm H_2O. The head of the bed should be elevated to 30° to protect the lungs from aspiration. Full cardiac monitoring must be used to titrate the administration of fluids, in order to avoid hypovolaemia or fluid overload and to minimise the unnecessary use of inotropic/pressor drugs. Urine output must be monitored and maintained at 0.5–2.5 ml/kg/hour. Incidences of diabetes insipidus are common and should be treated to maintain a blood glucose level of 4–8 mmol/litre. All electrolyte abnormalities must be corrected to as near to normal values as possible. Thromboprophylaxis is continued to prevent pulmonary emboli. Investigations requested by the retrieval team may include echocardiogram, bronchoscopy, virology screening, and HIV, Hep B and C if indicated. The administration of a 15 mg/kg of methylprednisolone is given to mediate the systemic inflammatory response associated with brain stem death. The continuation of all of these supportive measures should be maintained throughout the surgical phase of the organ retrieval until such time as they are no longer required.

4 **How would you prepare the theatre for the retrieval process?**

A The retrieval process is often undertaken at night when resources allow for a free theatre that does not interrupt an elective operating list, although this may have to be done in order not to delay the retrieval process. The preparation of the theatre environment is usually undertaken by a member of the theatre team. The theatre coordinator will be asked to provide a member of staff to circulate and a suitable theatre that is available and well stocked. Basic items such as an operating table, an anaesthetic machine, multiple suction units, drip stands, trolleys, Mayo stand, soft pack items, patient under-body warming blanket and a defibrillator with internal cardiac paddles may be required and should be available. The retrieval team will bring most of the specialised equipment, fluids and drugs with them, along with any items particular to the individual surgeons. They will usually require instrument trays such as a major laparotomy tray, minor basic tray, arterial tray, ice to pack the organs, 15+ litres of normal saline, UW solution (intracellular preservation solution), ligating clips, retractors for the abdomen, a sternal saw and retractor, vascular clamps, staplers and reloads, and sometimes a bronchoscope (NHSBT, 2014).

5 **What anaesthetic care do you think will be required in the retrieval procedure, and what is the rationale for these interventions?**

A Cardiovascular stability and ventilation for Mr Johnston after brain death (DBD) will be provided by either an anaesthetist who is part of the retrieval team, a donor care practitioner (DCP) or sometimes by the anaesthetist at the retrieval hospital. For donors after circulatory death (DCD) there is no requirement for anaesthetic or ventilatory support (McKeown *et al.*, 2012). While anaesthesia is not necessary, low concentrations of volatile agents are often used to treat hypertension and may have beneficial pre-conditioning effects. The criterion applied in the UK confirms unsurvivability by testing for brain stem death, and not for cerebral cortex death as they do in other countries. Therefore, if the cortex survives, then the use of a volatile agent seems compassionate. Adequate neuromuscular blockade to negate spinal reflex movements is required throughout the surgery (McKeown *et al.*, 2012).

6   **Consider the transfer to theatre. Who will attend this transfer and what would you need to consider when collecting Mr Johnston from the ICU?**

A   When all arrangements with the retrieval teams were in place, Mr Johnston's family said goodbye to him on the unit prior to his transfer to theatre. He was accompanied by the critical care nurse, the specialist nurse in organ donation, the on-call ODP and on-call anaesthetic registrar. He was transferred from the ICU bed on to the operating table and was connected to the anaesthetic machine; the retrieval anaesthetist then inserted a pulmonary artery catheter.

7   **What does the surgical procedure for organ retrieval involve?**

A   Surgical preparation for organ retrieval is as stringent and important as for any surgical procedure. The scrub team will be required to prepare themselves and their equipment using full aseptic technique and will maintain the sterile field throughout the procedure. The skin was prepared and shaved before being cleaned with a suitable surgical skin preparation agent. Draping then took place according to the surgeon's requirements for access. A midline incision from the suprasternal notch to the symphisis pubis was made to allow for access to all the abdominal and chest organs.

    The abdominal team performed a laparotomy to exclude any previously undiagnosed disease before dissection of the organs commenced. Initial mobilisation of the liver was undertaken, and identification and preservation of the inferior vena cava (IVC) and left hepatic artery was made. The common bile duct was ligated and divided before the gall bladder was opened; all of the bile removed and the biliary tree was flushed with cold saline. After mobilisation of the caecum, right colon and small bowel mesentery the distal IVC and abdominal aorta were exposed. The distal abdominal aorta was isolated and prepared for cannulation as was the inferior mesenteric vein. The descending thoracic aorta was also isolated and prepared for cross-clamping.

    Mobilisation of the kidneys was undertaken at this point, although they were left in situ for removal at the end of the procedure. The cardiac team then made an assessment of the intrathoracic organs and decided to proceed. The superior vena cava (SVC) and IVC were isolated, and the ascending aorta cannulated. At this point the donor patient was given 20,000 IU heparin. Cannulation of the descending aorta to perfuse the abdominal organs and the inferior mesenteric vein to perfuse the liver followed. The aorta was then cross-clamped, and perfusion of the heart and abdominal organs commenced. The IVC was incised below the pericardium, and the heart and liver were allowed to empty. The pericardial sac and the abdominal cavity were filled with cold saline (4°C) and slush sterile ice. Cold UW (University of Wisconsin) solution was then perfused via the cannulae into the organs. UW solution was developed in the 1980s to preserve the intracellular structure of donated organs. A cardioplegic solution containing potassium and glucose was used to arrest and cool the heart. This protects the myocardium by inducing a rapid and complete diastolic arrest, minimising myocardial energy requirements and preventing ischaemic damage (Smith, 2003). The heart was then removed and placed on ice into a sterile bowl. Ventilation was continued until the lungs were perfused via the pulmonary artery with the preservation solution and the trachea had been stapled with the lungs fully inflated. The liver, pancreas and kidneys were then removed with their accessory vessels intact. All organs were preserved in UW solution. Lymph nodes and sections of the spleen were removed to provide cells for tissue typing.

When the major organs had been removed and packed appropriately they were then placed into the care of the specialist nurse in organ donation, who coordinated the transfer of the organs to the appropriate donor centres. The abdominal surgical team closed the chest and abdomen with a silk suture and covered the wound with a surgical dressing. No tendons were removed and corneal retrieval was undertaken in the mortuary. The drapes were removed, and Mr Johnston was cleaned and transferred to the post-anaesthetic care unit (PACU).

8 **What care interventions are undertaken in the postoperative period?**

A Last offices are often undertaken as part of the postoperative care of the patient undergoing organ donation. It is important that any cultural or religious views are considered during this process and these should form the basis of any care given, alongside any relevant local policy. Mr Johnston was not a religious man and his family did not make any special requirements with regard to last offices. A non-denominational last offices procedure was carried out in line with the trust hospital policy by the critical care nurse, the theatre practitioner present during the procedure and the specialist nurse in organ donation in the PACU. The family did not wish to view the body before removal to the hospital mortuary.

Stop and think

While Mr Johnston was not religious and there were no specific requests regarding last offices, consider how familiar you are with the requirements of different religions. It is important to have an understanding of these as they do have a significant impact upon how perioperative patients are cared for once deceased, so find out the main requirements of different religions.

---

9 **What information do you think Mr Johnston's family may want following the retrieval process?**

A Post-retrieval care is focused on the organ donor's family and friends. The specialist nurse in organ donation can facilitate correspondence between donating and receiving families. Knowing that donated organs have helped other people live can be a significant factor in helping people come to terms with the loss of a loved one. Mr Johnston was on the UK donor register and carried a donor card. As a family they had previously discussed donation and were in full support of the donation of his organs. Afterwards the family received confirmation from the specialist nurse in organ donation that had worked alongside the critical care and theatre teams that Mr Johnston's organs had helped five people, and subsequent correspondence that they sent in to the ICU said that they found this to be a huge comfort to the whole family.

10   **Why is it important to improve wider communications and discussion relating to organ donation?**

A   Although it is a complex and emotive process, organ transplantation offers many people with end-stage organ failure the only hope of improved quality of life, freedom from lifelong treatment regimes and is often their only hope of improved survival. By improving communication, and by implementing a multidisciplinary approach to the identification, referral and management of potential organ donors, the aim is to close the gap between the number of available organs and those who are waiting for a transplant, and to reduce the number of people dying daily while waiting for a transplant.

Stop and think

Organ donation is an emotive topic and different people have many different experiences and thoughts related to this. Try to consider these different perspectives and why it is important to be aware of these to care for the patient and their family.

Also consider how the theatre team may feel following the retrieval procedure and last offices. Where can support be obtained if someone feels that they need it?

REFERENCES AND FURTHER READING

Cota, N., Burgess, M. and English, W. (2013) Organ donation after circulatory death. Available online at: www.totw.anaesthesiologists.org (accessed 8 March 2014).

McKeown, D., Bonser, R. and Kellum, J. (2012) Management of the heartbeating brain-dead organ donor. *British Journal of Anaesthesia*, **108**: 96–107.

National Institute for Health and Clinical Excellence (NICE) (2011) *Organ Donation for Transplantation: Improving Donor Identification and Consent Rates for Deceased Organ Donation*. London: NICE.

NHS Blood and Transplant (NHSBT) (2013) *National Standards for Organ Retrieval from Deceased Donors*. London: National Health Service.

NHS Blood and Transplant (NHSBT) (2014) *Abdominal Perfusion and Preservation Protocols for NORS Teams in the UK*. London: National Health Service.

Smith, S. (2003) Organ and tissue donation and recovery. *Organ Transplant*, **3**: 1–16.

Wessels, T., Moller-Hartmann, W., Noth, J. and Klotzsch, C. (2004) CT findings and clinical features as markers for patient outcome in primary pontine haemorrhage. *American Journal of Neuroradiology*, **25**: 257–260.

Index

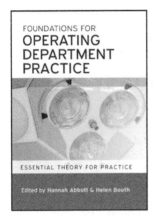

FOUNDATIONS FOR OPERATING DEPARTMENT PRACTICE
Essential theory for practice

Abbott and Booth

ISBN: 9780335244973 (Paperback)
eISBN: 9780335244980

2014

Foundations for Operating Department Practice is written specifically by Operating Department Practitioners (ODPs) for Operating Department Practitioners, and is the first book of its kind to bring together the fundamental professional knowledge that supports and underpins the ODP's practice to enable them to deliver effective, compassionate and evidence-based care to the patient. This new text supports pre and post-registration Operating Department Practitioners throughout their academic studies and beyond in their professional careers, encapsulating the attributes needed in the unique context of the ODP profession. It covers:

- Working in the Perioperative Team
- Research and Evidence-Based Practice
- Patient Safety
- Psychosocial Aspects of Operating Department Practice
- Ethics and Legal Frameworks
- Reflection, Leadership and Management
- Professional Practice, Lifelong Learning and Continued Professional Development

www.mheducation.co.uk

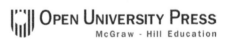

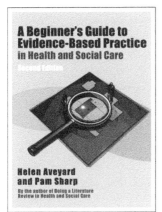

A BEGINNER'S GUIDE TO EVIDENCE-BASED
PRACTICE IN HEALTH AND SOCIAL CARE

Second Edition

Helen Aveyard and Pam Sharp

ISBN: 9780335246724 (Paperback)
eBook:

2013

**Have you heard of 'evidence based practice' but don't know what it
means?**
Are you having trouble relating evidence to your practice?

This is **the** book for anyone who has ever wondered what evidence based
practice is or how to relate it to practice. Fully updated in this brand new
edition, this book is simple and easy to understand – and designed to help
those new to the topic to apply the concept to their practice and learning
with ease.

Key features:

- Additional material on literature reviews and searching for literature
- Even more examples for health and social care practice
- Extra material on qualitative research and evidence based practice
- Expanded section on hierarchies of evidence and how to use them

www.mheducation.co.uk

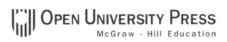

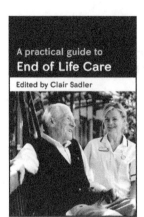

A Practical guide to End of Life Care

Sadler

ISBN: 9780335263561 (Paperback)
eISBN: 9780335263578

2015

Are you involved in caring for people at the end of their life? Do you have a role in supporting the families of those who are dying, or is this an area of your work you find personally difficult?

This book is an accessible guide for all those working in health or social care and caring for people at the end of their lives. Written for healthcare assistants, hospice workers, volunteers, nurses and other carers, the book will prove an essential source of guidance and support for those working in the community, care homes, hospices, hospitals or other settings.

Easy-to-read chapters emphasize treating people who are dying with dignity, using a person-centred approach. The authors promote quality care by recognizing physical and non-physical symptoms, and the emotional and physical needs people might have. Advice is also given about the importance of care givers' well-being.

Written by experts with extensive experience in delivering high quality end of life care, this book is full of tips from real life practice, reflection exercises and case studies. It also includes insights into what can help make a good death, and how to help support families at the end of life.

www.mheducation.co.uk

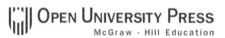

OPEN UNIVERSITY PRESS
McGraw - Hill Education

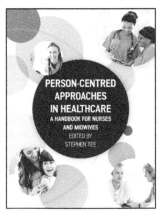

Person-centred approaches in healthcare
A handbook for nurses and midwives

Tee

ISBN: 9780335263585 (Paperback)
eISBN: 9780335263592

2016

Written by practitioners, academics and, more importantly, the people who use health services, this unique text examines the application of person-centred principles across a range of healthcare contexts. It will provide you with the essential skills, techniques and strategies needed to deliver person-centred care.

Patients and service users should be at the heart of healthcare delivery and this book will equip nurses and midwives by connecting the reader to the lived experience of those receiving healthcare. It examines issues across the lifespan and reveals how person-centred care can best be achieved by working in partnership.

After introducing key principles and service design in chapters 1 and 2, each chapter that follows tackles a different age or disease specific area of care, including:

- Maternity care
- Family care including health visiting
- Adolescent care
- Adult critical care
- Diseases including diabetes and arthritis
- Care for people with long term mental health problems
- Intellectual disabilities
- Care of carers

www.mheducation.co.uk

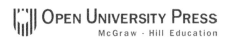